EAT SO WHAT!
THE POWER OF VEGETARIANISM

Nutrition Guide for Weight Loss, Disease Free, Drug Free, Healthy Long Life (Full Version)

Revised and updated

LA FONCEUR

Copyright © 2019 La Fonceur

All rights reserved.

ISBN 978-1-09777-377-0

This book has been published with all efforts taken to make the material error-free. The information on this book is not intended or implied to be a substitute for diagnosis, prognosis, treatment, prescription, and/or dietary advice from a licensed health professional. Author doesn't assume and hereby disclaim any liability to any party for any loss, damage, or disruption caused by errors or omissions, whether such errors or omissions result from negligence, accident, or any other cause.

While every effort has been made to avoid any mistake or omission, this publication is being sold on the condition and understanding that neither the author nor the publishers or printers would be liable in any manner to any person by reason of any mistake or omission in this publication or for any action taken or omitted to be taken or advice rendered or accepted on the basis of this work.

Get rid of Anemia, Vitamin B12 Deficiency, and Protein Deficiency with Eat So What! The Power of Vegetarianism.

- La Fonceur

CONTENTS

Preface	7
CHAPTER 1	9
What are Nutrients? Why are They So Important?	9
CHAPTER 2	21
Top 10 Health Benefits of Being a Vegetarian	21
CHAPTER 3	31
10 Reasons You Should Eat More Protein Every Day	31
CHAPTER 4	40
10 High Protein Sources for Vegetarians	40
CHAPTER 5	49
10 Reasons Why Fat is Not the Enemy. The Truth About Fats!	49
CHAPTER 6	61
Top 10 Healthy Fat Foods You Should Eat	61
CHAPTER 7	72
10 Reasons You Should Never Give Up Carbohydrates	72
CHAPTER 8	82
10 Healthy Carbohydrates You Must Eat for Health and Nutrition Benefits	82
Preventive Measures	95

CHAPTER 9

10 Power Foods to Get Rid of Anemia   **97**

CHAPTER 10

Top 10 Foods for Vegetarians to Prevent Vitamin B12 Deficiency   **107**

CHAPTER 11

Recipes   **115**

   Chilli Tofu   117

   Beans in Schezwan Sauce   120

   Mushroom Fried Pulao   122

   Khajur Roll   125

About the Author   **128**

Note from La Fonceur   **129**

All Books by La Fonceur   **130**

Connect with La Fonceur   **131**

Preface

Being a Lacto Vegetarian, I always look for healthy vegetarian options to include in my diet. Everyone's body is different. Everyone reacts differently to food. Some are allergic to nuts, some have a naturally weak immune system. In this book, I have included food options that everyone can include in their diet.

I see various diet trends catching fire every day, but these are far from being a healthy diet. These diets may give a temporary solution for health issues, whether it is obesity, diabetes, or other diseases. But for healthy living, one must have a thorough knowledge of foods that they eat, the actual purpose of foods, and how nutritious they are.

In *Eat So What! The Power of Vegetarianism*, you are going to understand your food scientifically and realistically. Do not be misled by any random diet. Learn why each nutrient is important. How can you get maximum health benefits from nutrients when you choose the right type. Learn how to prevent anemia, vitamin B12, and protein deficiency while you are vegetarian.

When you include the right nutrients in the right amount in your diet, you don't need supplements. Learn how you can practice vegetarianism all naturally without any human-made supplements.

Whether you are vegetarian since birth or practicing vegetarianism for health issues or a non-vegetarian, *Eat So What! The Power of Vegetarianism* book is for you.

Being a Research Scientist and Registered Pharmacist, I have worked closely with drugs, and based on my experience, I would suggest not to depend on drugs but to eat healthy vegetarian foods that have the power to protect you from many diseases. Vegetarian diet can add valuable and healthy years to your life. In this book, I am throwing light on the fact that how plant-based healthy vegetarian foods are the remedy to most of our daily health problems.

You will also discover some tasty and healthy recipes to boost your health as well as satisfy your urge to eat out. Discover some simple yet recipes that anyone can cook at home. You no longer need to compromise on taste to eat healthy foods.

La Fonceur

CHAPTER 1

What are Nutrients? Why are They So Important?

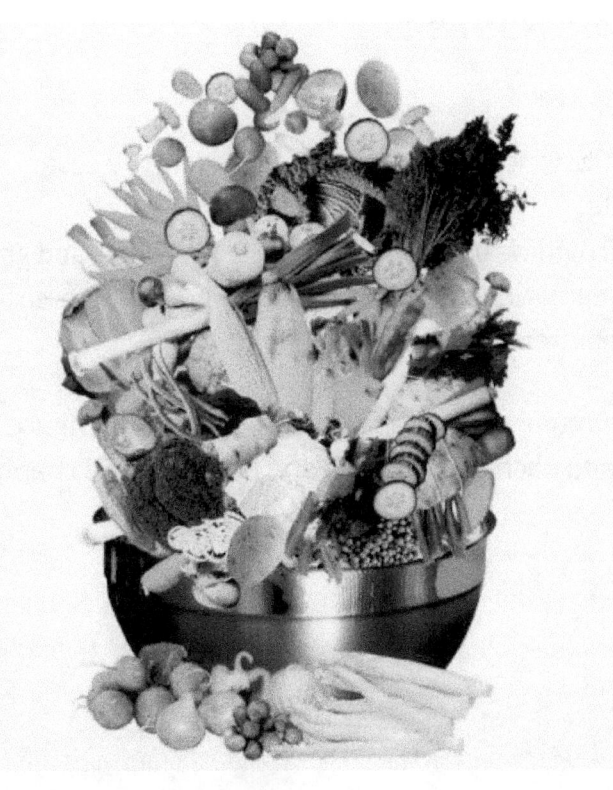

N utrients are this, nutrients are that, falla food is more nutritious, falla food should not be eaten as it is not nutritious, blah blah blah... you may have heard these things thousands of times. So many fuss about nutrition value, but the question is, what factors decide which food is more nutritious and which one is not? What makes food nutritious? The Answer is, the number of nutrients present in a food decides its nutrition value. Now, what are Nutrients?

This chapter will answer all of your questions about nutrients.

What are Nutrients?

Nutrients are:

- Substances present in our food and are essential for our life.
- Providing us energy, essential for repair and growth.
- Regulating chemical processes, and necessary for the maintenance of overall health.

I have summarised all about nutrients in the figure. We will understand each one in detail one by one in this chapter.

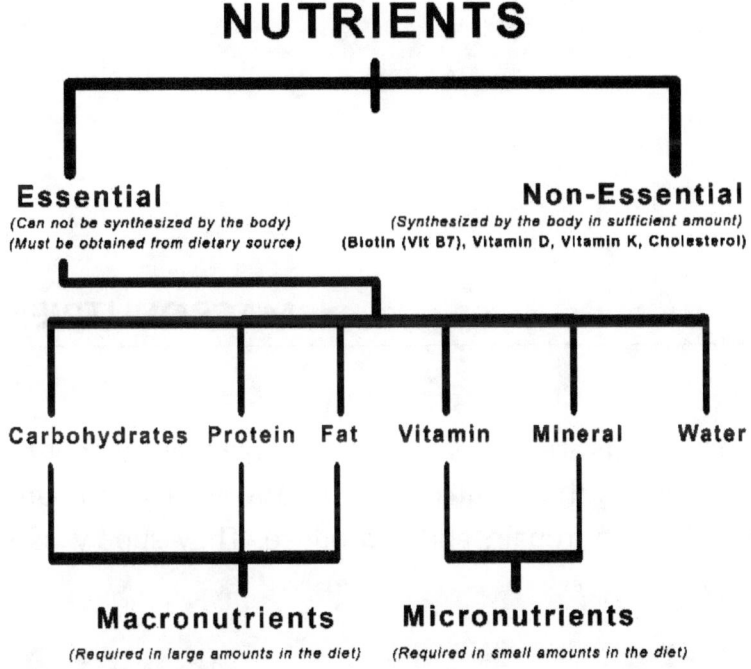

Types of Nutrients:

Essential nutrients

Nonessential nutrients

ESSENTIAL NUTRIENTS

Essential nutrients either cannot be synthesized by the body or synthesized in insufficient quantity and are required for normal body functioning thus must be obtained from foods.

Essential nutrients are divided into 2 parts:

Macronutrients

Micronutrients

MACRONUTRIENTS

Macronutrients are the main nutrients that make up our foods. Body requires these nutrients in relatively large amounts to grow, develop, repair, and reproduce. They supply us with energy.

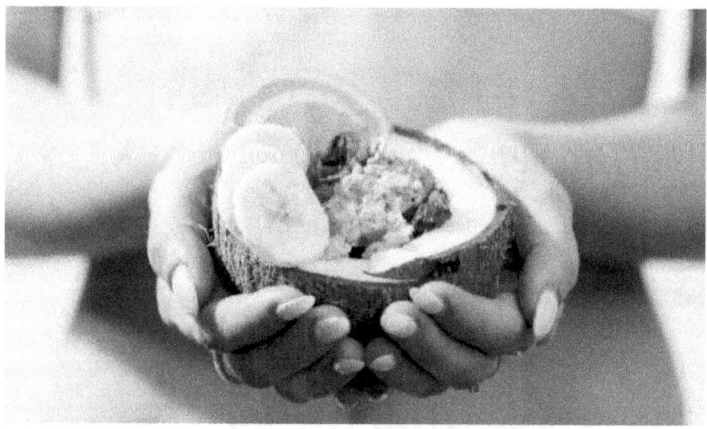

The three macronutrients are carbohydrate, protein, and fat, with the fourth bonus, water. All these three macronutrients have their own specific functions in the body. Almost every food has all of the macronutrients, but foods are classified based on the highest percentage of macronutrient present in it. For example, a coconut consists up of 50% fat, 10% carbohydrates, and 6% protein, so this would be classified as fat, while a banana consists of 80% carbohydrates, with only small amounts of protein and fats, so this would be classified as a carbohydrate.

1. *Carbohydrates*

By definition, carbohydrates cannot be listed as essential macronutrients as the body can synthesize all the carbohydrates on its own, but it is recommended to get most of the energy from carbohydrates. Therefore, they are required in relatively large amounts for normal body functioning, and carbohydrates are a healthy nutrient choice.

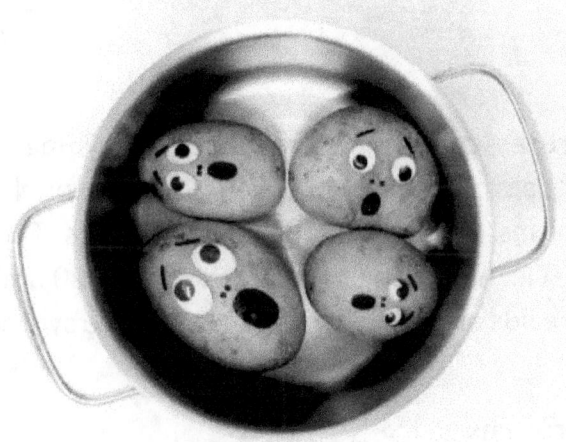

Carbohydrates are comprised of small chains of sugar that break down into glucose by enzyme salivary amylase present in our mouth to use as the body's primary energy source and therefore needs to make up around 50-65% of a diet. Carbohydrates are important in supplying energy to the brain, improving digestion, playing key roles in development, supporting normal immune function, preventing pathogenesis and blood clotting.

2. Proteins

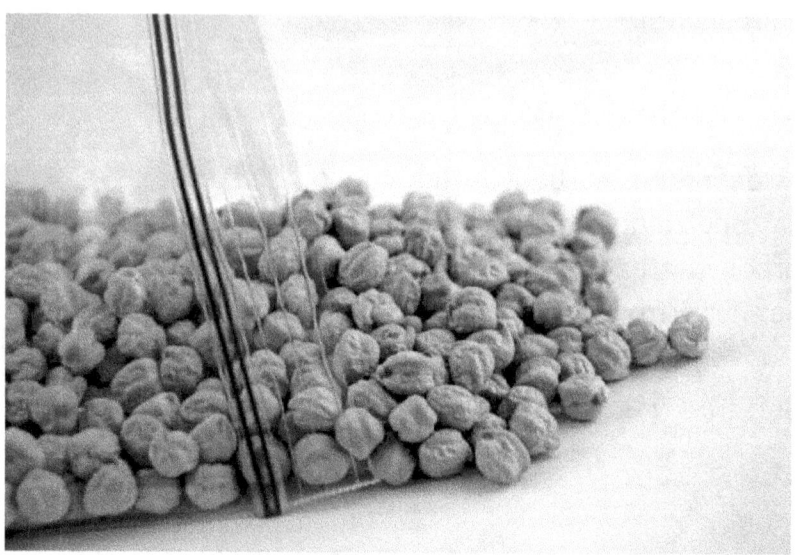

Proteins are essential macronutrients, consisting of one or more long chain of amino acid which is the essential part of all living organisms, especially as the building blocks of body tissue such as muscle, hair, bones, nails, etc. Among 20 amino acids, nine amino acids are essential which cannot be synthesized by the body.

Essential Proteins:

- Histidine
- Isoleucine
- Leucine
- Lysine
- Methionine
- Phenylalanine

- Threonine
- Tryptophan
- Valine

3. *Fat*

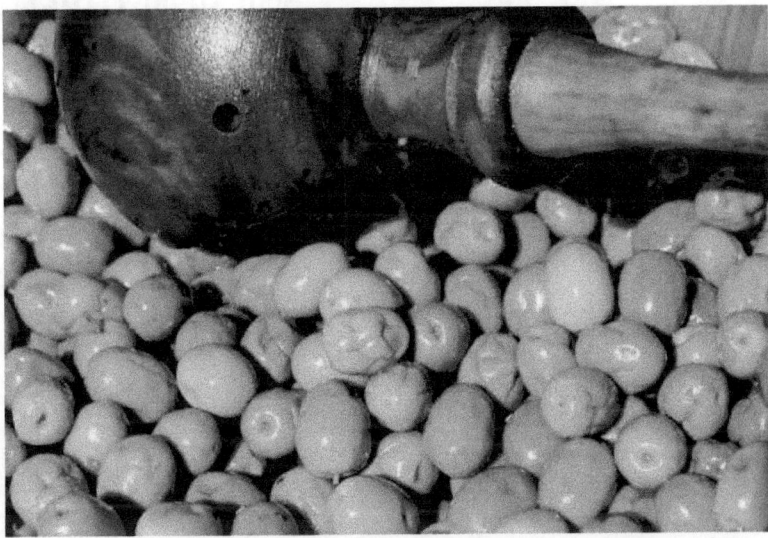

Fat is an essential nutrient and boosts absorption of fat-soluble vitamins such as Vitamin A, D, E, K and helps protect internal organs.

Essential Fatty Acids:
- Alpha-linolenic acid (omega-3 fatty acid)
- Linoleic acid (omega-6 fatty acid)

MICRONUTRIENTS

Micronutrients are required in small amounts, but they are just as vital as macronutrients for normal body functioning. Micronutrients support metabolism and enable the body to produce hormones, enzymes, and other substances essential for proper growth and development.

Types of micronutrients:

Vitamins

MInerals

Vitamins

Vitamins are organic compounds. Humans require thirteen vitamins in their diet. Vitamins are classified as either water-soluble (vitamin B Complex and vitamin C) or fat-soluble (A, D, E, and K). Water-soluble vitamins get dissolve in water and are readily excreted from the body. This is why a consistent intake of water-soluble vitamins is required. Fat-soluble vitamins require lipid in the body to be absorbed through the intestinal tract.

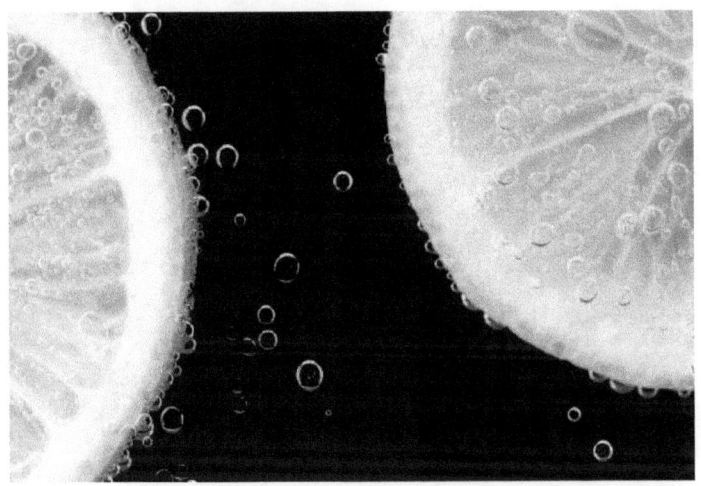

Vitamins act as coenzymes or cofactors for various proteins, which are part of many chemical reactions in the body. Vitamin A is vital for healthy skin, teeth, mucus membranes, and eyes. Vitamin C for immunity. Vitamin D absorbs calcium to promote bone growth and cardiovascular health. Vitamin B6 helps form red blood cells and maintain brain function.

Essential Vitamins:

Fat-soluble vitamins

Water-soluble vitamins

Fat-soluble Vitamins are

- Vitamin A
- Vitamin D
- Vitamin E
- Vitamin K

Water-soluble Vitamins are

- Vitamin B Complex

- Thiamine (Vitamin B1)
- Riboflavin (Vitamin B2)
- Niacin (Vitamin B3)
- Pantothenic acid (Vitamin B5)
- Pyroxidine (Vitamin B6)
- Biotin (Vitamin B7)
- Folate (Vitamin B9)
- Cobalamin (Vitamin B12)
* Vitamin C

Vitamin B7 and Vitamin D can be synthesized by the body but in insufficient quantity.

Minerals

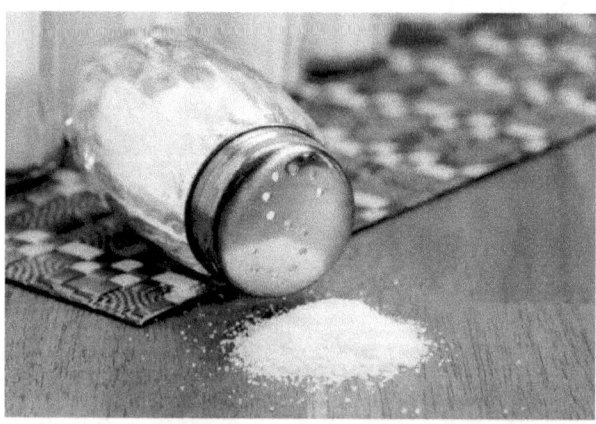

Minerals are inorganic and retain their chemical structure. Minerals are mainly needed for metabolism. They are important for healthy bones, muscle contraction, proper fluid balance, and nerve transmission in the body.

Essential Minerals:

Major Minerals

- Calcium
- Sodium
- Potassium
- Magnesium
- Phosphorus

Trace Minerals

- Iodine
- Iron
- Zinc
- Copper
- Chlorine
- Sulfur
- Manganese
- Cobalt
- Molybdenum
- Selenium

NONESSENTIAL NUTRIENTS

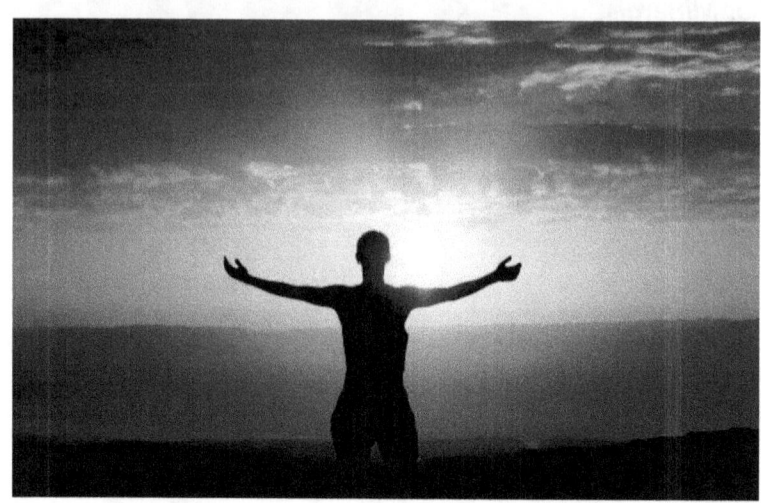

Nonessential nutrients can be synthesized by the body in sufficient quantity or obtained from sources other than foods.

Some examples of Nonessential nutrients:

- Biotin or Vitamin B7 is produced by gastrointestinal bacteria.
- Vitamin K is produced by intestinal bacteria present in the colon.
- Vitamin D is produced by the body when the skin is exposed to sunlight.
- Cholesterol is produced by the liver in a good amount. This is the reason you don't need to add extra cholesterol to your diet.

CHAPTER 2

Top 10 Health Benefits of Being a Vegetarian

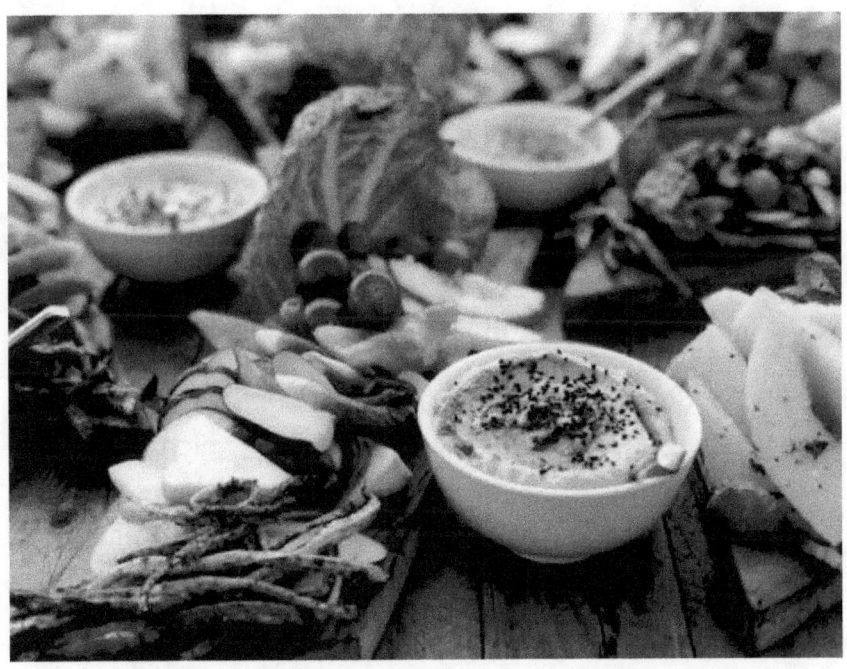

What is Vegetarianism?

Vegetarianism is the practice of abstaining from the consumption of animal products, including red meat, fish or other seafood, poultry, the flesh of animals, or byproducts of animal slaughter. A vegetarian diet includes grains, fruits, vegetables, pulses, nuts, seeds, and with or without dairy products and eggs.

There are different types of vegetarians:

- **Lacto-vegetarians** exclude animal products and eggs but eat dairy products.

- **Lacto-ovo-vegetarians** exclude animal products but eat both dairy products and eggs.

- **Jain vegetarians** exclude animal products, eggs, or anything that grows underground, including potatoes, onions, and garlic but eat dairy products.

- **Buddhist vegetarians** exclude animal products and vegetables in the allium family (which have the characteristic aroma of onion and garlic): onion, garlic, chives, scallions, leeks, or shallots but eat dairy products.

- **Vegans** exclude any products derived from animals – no meat, fish, dairy, or eggs.

*Read 10 Nutrient Combinations You Should Eat for Maximum Health Benefits in the book Eat to Prevent and Control Disease.

Below are the top 10 health benefits of being a vegetarian:

1. Slows the Aging Process, Increases Lifespan

Vegetarian organic plant-based diet is mainly rich in vitamins and minerals, antioxidants, phytonutrients, and fiber, which in turn strengthens the immune system. It flushes out toxins from the body, prevents chemical build-up in the body that slows down the aging process.

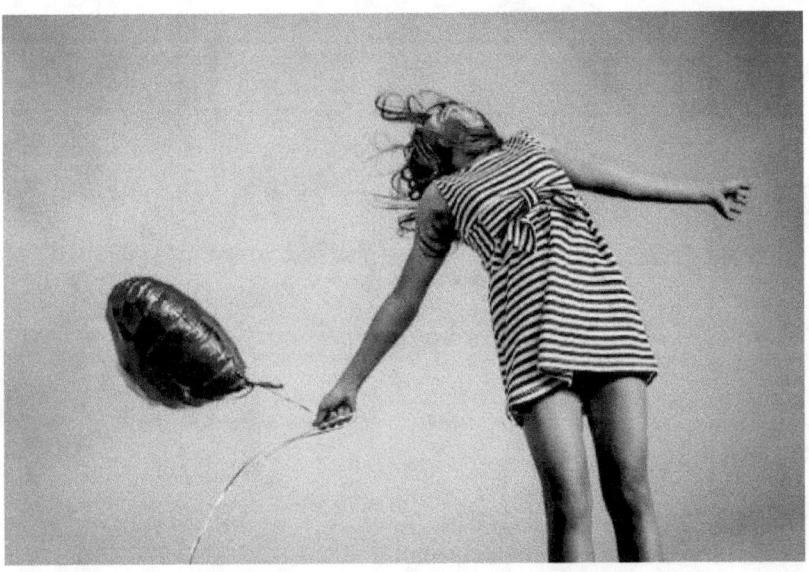

Additionally, a vegetarian diet can prevent many chronic diseases, thus facilitating more healthy years and a longer lifespan.

2. Less Toxicity

Toxins such as pesticides, antibiotics, hormones are all fat-soluble. They concentrate on the fatty flesh of the animals. Non-vegetarian foods can harbor contaminants such viruses and parasites such as toxoplasmosis parasites, Trichinella spiralis, salmonella, and other worms. Food-borne illnesses, bacteria, and chemical toxins are more common in commercial meat, seafood, and poultry than in organic plant-based foods.

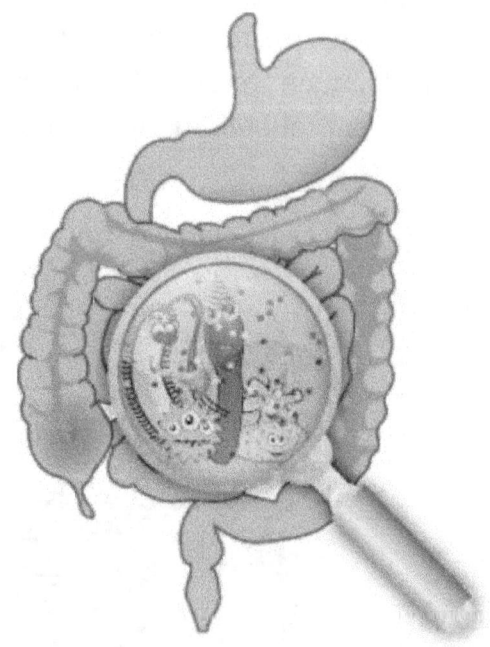

3. Improves Metabolism

Fiber is necessary for proper digestion. Fruits and vegetables contain high fiber content. Vegetarian food is easy to digest and helps in the fast elimination of toxins and other chemicals from the body, keeping the body metabolism in a good state. RMR (resting metabolic rate) in people with a vegetarian diet is higher than omnivores which means vegetarians speedily burn fats.

4. Maintains Healthy Body Weight

Typically, Vegetarians weigh less. Vegetarians usually have a lower body mass index (a measure of body fat) than meat-eaters. This may be because a vegetarian diet typically comprises fewer calories and high in fiber, such as vegetables and fruits, grains, legumes, nuts, and seeds that are more filling, lower in fat, and less calorie-dense. This might be the main reason why more and more people today are opting for vegetarianism in their life.

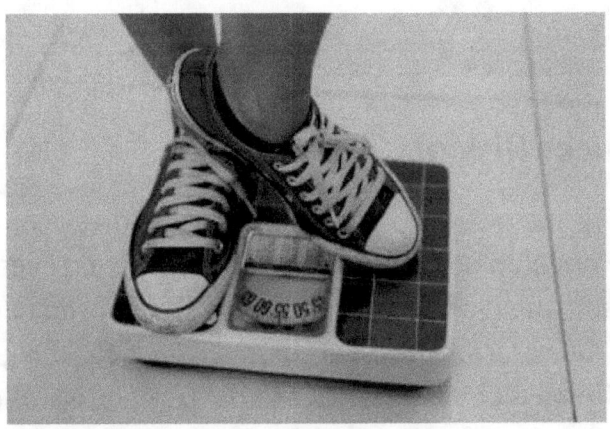

5. Reduces Risk of Diabetes

As per a study, diabetes is more frequently occurs in Non-vegetarians almost twice as often as in vegetarians. A vegetarian diet provides greater protection against diabetes. Healthy vegetarian diets are easy to absorb, contain less fatty acids, and more nutritious. Vegetarian diets are beneficial in Type 2 diabetes, where weight loss is the most effective way to manage the condition.

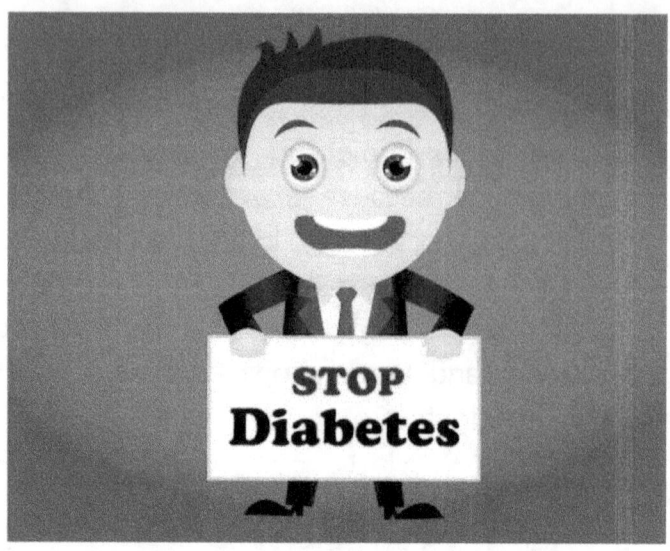

6. Reduces Risk of Cataract

Though it cannot be confirmed that eating meat causes cataract development, but many studies have revealed that decreases in meat consumption as part of a daily diet decreases the risk for cataracts. Researchers suggest that vegetarians' overall lifestyle contributes to the decreased risk of cataract, and vegetarians enjoy less incidence of cataract development.

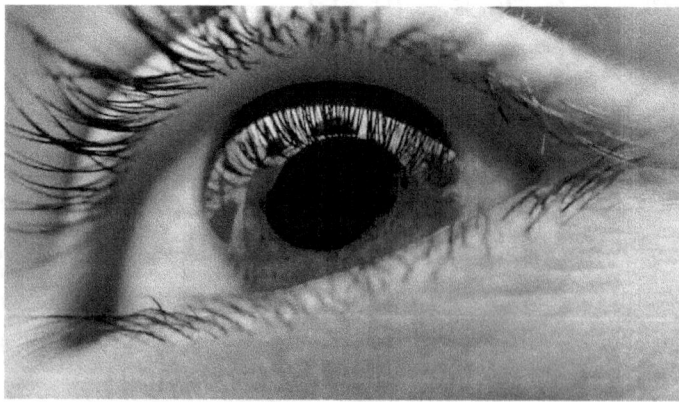

7. Reduces Risk of Cancer

Red meat and processed meat consumption are directly associated with an increase in the risk of colorectal cancer. There is evidence that vegetarians have a statistically significantly lower cancer rate than those who consume meat regularly. A vegetarian diet contains fruits and vegetables that are high in antioxidants which protect against cancer. Reducing your risk of cancer is another great reason to opt for vegetarianism.

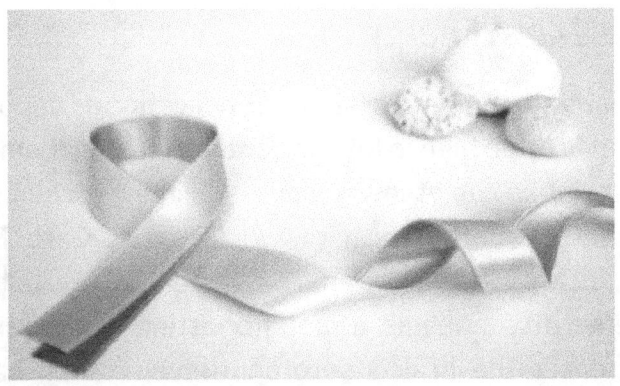

8. Reduces Risk of Heart Disease

Vegetarian diets are rich in fiber, antioxidants, and phytonutrients, which are known to reduce oxidative stress and inflammation, which may support a significantly reduced risk of heart disease. Also, Vegetarian diets are lower in saturated fat and cholesterol than meat-based diets that are often high in cholesterol, fat, and environmental pollutants. Vegetarians have a 40 percent less risk of death from cardiovascular disease than non-vegetarians.

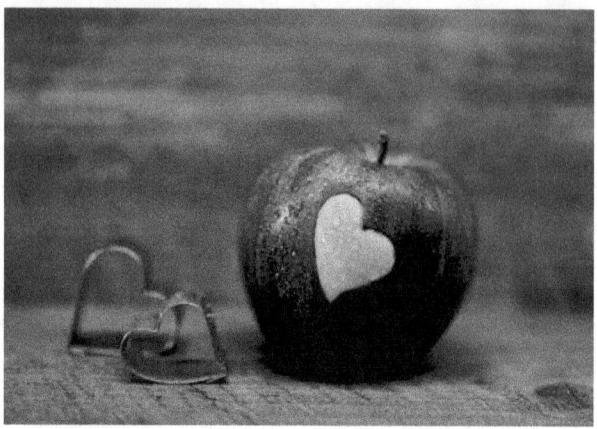

9. Gives More Energy

Vegetarians are tending to be more energetic and happy. Meat-based diet is often high in fat and protein, making them difficult to digest, while vegetarians have a higher consumption of carbohydrates in the form of whole grain. Carbohydrates digest quickly and give energy instantly. Carbohydrates increase serotonin levels, a mood-boosting neurotransmitter that increases the brain's serotonin levels called happiness hormones which keep you happy all day.

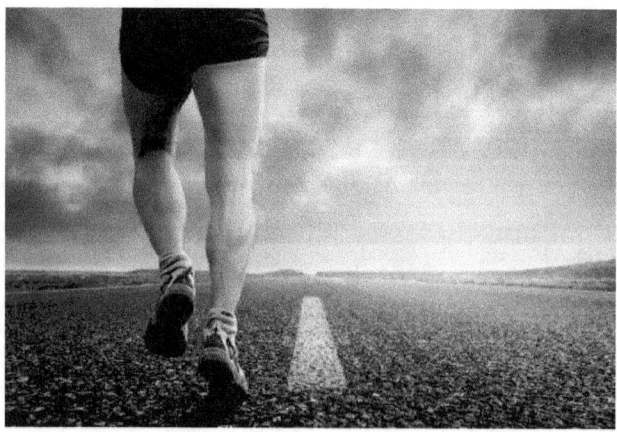

10. Lowers Cholesterol Levels

Vegetarian diet is much low in cholesterol, while animal products are very high in cholesterol. High levels of LDL cholesterol (low-density lipoprotein - bad cholesterol) have been linked with an increased risk of coronary heart disease (CHD).

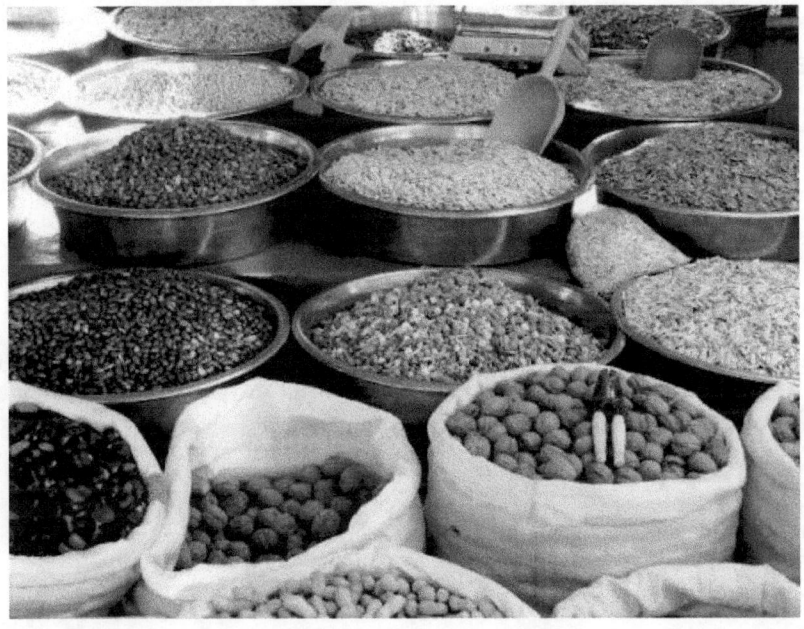

Vegetarian diets are associated with lower cholesterol levels. This may be because vegetarians have reduced intake of saturated fat, and an increased intake of organic plant-based foods, like fruits, vegetables, whole grains, legumes, seeds, and nuts that are naturally rich in soluble fiber, protein, and plant sterols. Although cholesterol is an essential component of human cell, there is no need to take cholesterol from an external source. Our body can make all the cholesterol it needs from vegetarian foods.

Conclusion

Along with a healthy organic vegetarian diet, many other factors contribute to a healthy and long lifespan. Some other lifestyle choices need to pay attention to, like quitting smoking and drinking. Being on a vegetarian diet doesn't mean you opt for less healthy food options, such as refined grains, which could increase the risk of heart disease. One should follow plant-based diets high in fiber, whole grains, vegetables, legumes, seeds, and nuts that are lower in fat, more filling, healthy and nutritious.

CHAPTER 3

10 Reasons You Should Eat More Protein Every Day

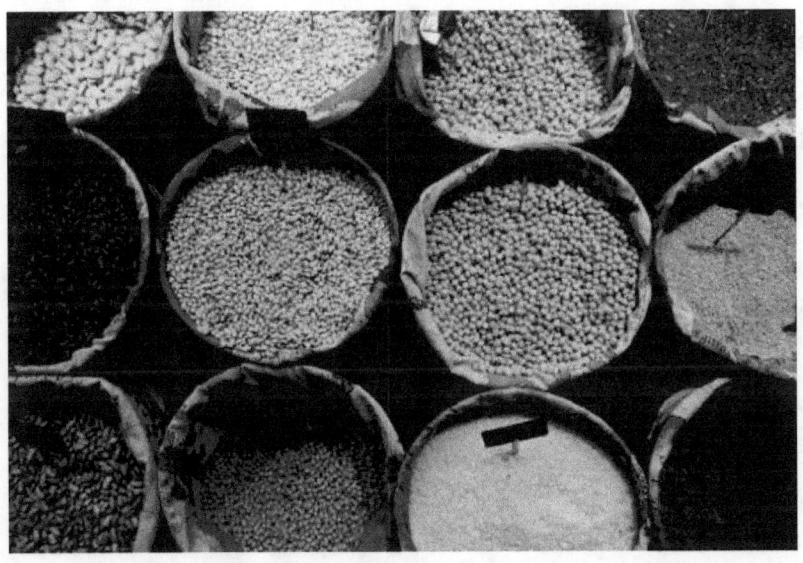

What is Protein?

Proteins are essential macronutrients, consisting of one or more long chain of amino acid which is the essential part of all living organisms, especially as the building blocks of body tissue such as muscle, hair, bones, nails, etc.

Daily Recommended Protein Amount

Recommended Dietary Allowances (RDA), the daily dietary intake level of a nutrient considered sufficient to meet your basic nutritional requirements. RDA for protein is 0.8 grams of protein per kilogram of body weight.

RDA is shown below for males and females aged 19-70 years:

Male: 56 g/day

Female: 46 g/day

Below are the 10 reasons you should eat more protein every day:

1. Anti-Aging

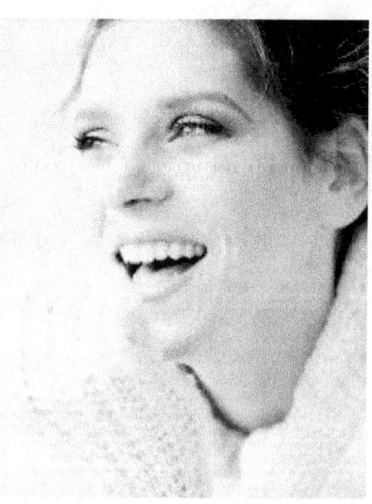

Wrinkles are caused primarily by sun damage and loss of the proteins- collagen and elastin. As we grow older, our body inevitably loses muscle mass. One of the easiest ways to improve your muscle mass and keep your body healthy is to follow a protein-rich diet that accelerates the healing and nourishing skin. Whey protein is good for anti-aging nutrition, contains branch chain amino acids that heal and nourish the skin and prevent signs of aging.

2. *Speeds Up Recovery from Injury*

Protein is an important building block of body tissues, including muscle. Protein can help the body repair after it has been injured and speeds up the recovery process. Protein digests into the amino acids which are required to repair damaged muscles. A steady supply of amino acids is needed to promote healing in the body. Protein helps to rebuild any lost muscle. Body needs extra protein post-injury. The protein-rich diet allows the body to produce new collagen and elastin to help keep tendons and ligaments strong.

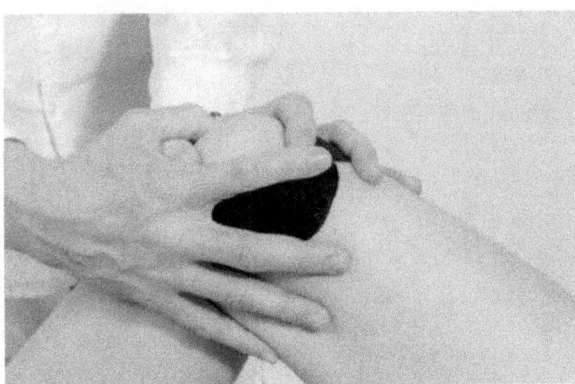

3. *Boost Muscle Mass*

Protein is the building block of muscles. Eating adequate amounts of protein promotes muscle growth and helps in maintaining muscle mass. To gain muscle mass, one should do exercise and strength training along with high rich protein diet. Also, the constant supply of protein throughout the day is essential for optimum muscle growth.

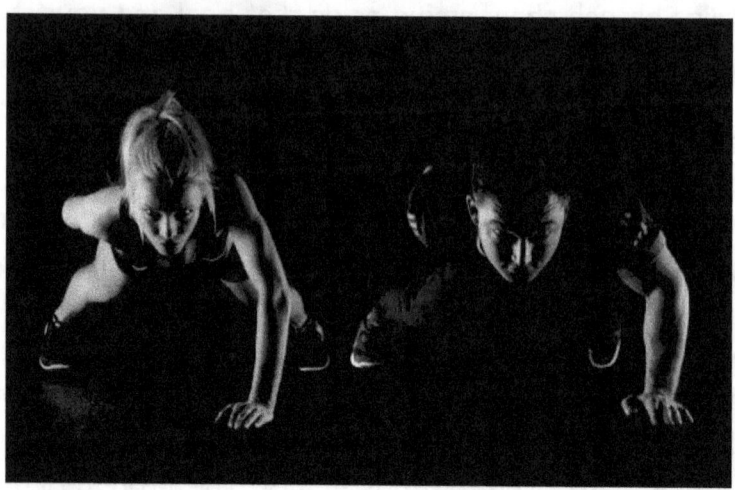

4. Healthy Skin

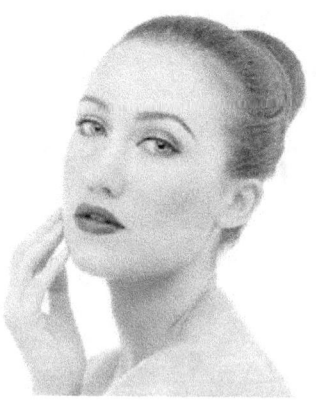

Protein is a building block of skin tissue. It is excellent for the general health of the skin and for its ability to repair itself. Protein breaks down into amino acids for the body's constant reconstruction job. Amino acids help construct collagen and create lubricating ceramide in the skin, keeping the skin healthy. It also repairs the skin-damaging done by the sun and environmental irritants.

5. Reduces Appetite, Increases Satiety

Protein helps you stay full for longer with less food. Eating a high-protein diet can boost the release of a hunger-suppressing hormone peptide. Because of the hormone peptide, you do not have cravings, and you control your hunger. Protein also reduces levels of appetite-spiking hormone ghrelin, so you don't get massive cravings at night. It makes you eat fewer calories automatically.

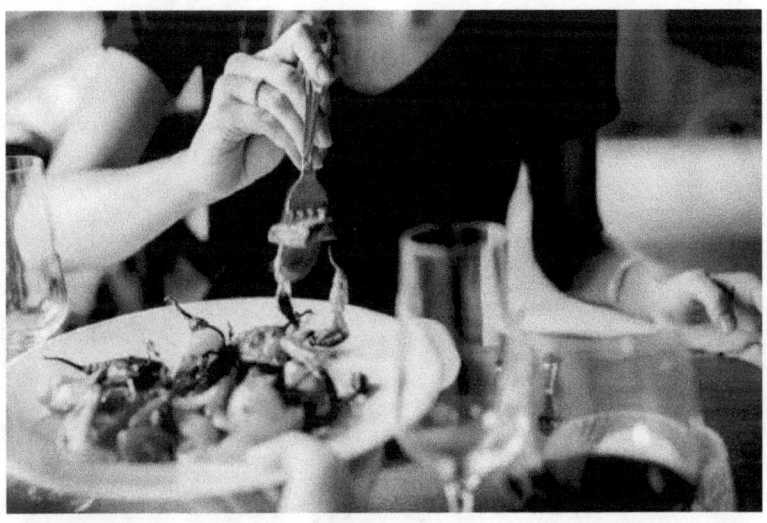

6. Burns More Calories

When you replace some of carbs and fats with protein in your diet, you actually burn more calories as protein boosts your metabolism. This is because our body needs some calories to digest and metabolize the food. The number of calories required to burn protein into fuel is much higher than fats and carbs. It means your body will burn more calories over the course of the day. This way, your metabolism will be more efficient, and you lose more weight.

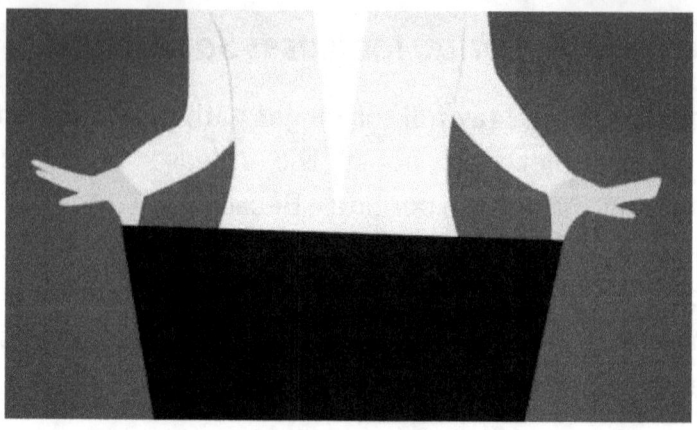

7. Controls Diabetes

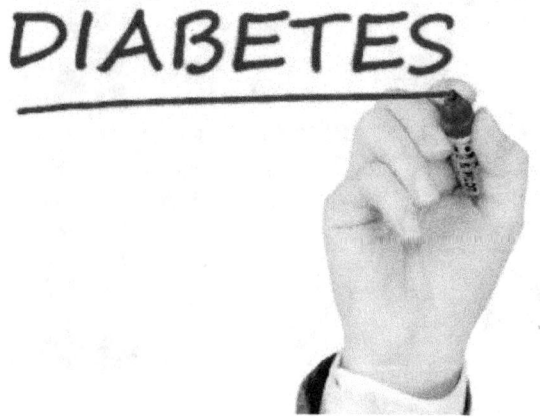

Diets high in protein and low in carbohydrates may help Type 2 diabetes patients improve their blood sugar levels. Protein breaks down into glucose less efficiently than carbohydrates and, as a result, takes longer to reach the bloodstream, cause insulin to release gradually, helping the body maintain healthy glucose levels.

Read in detail about how to prevent and control diabetes in the book Eat to Prevent and Control Disease.

8. Lowers Blood Pressure

Short-term clinical trials suggest that dietary protein lowers blood pressure. High-protein diets might reduce the risk of cardiovascular disease by lowering blood pressure. Higher protein diets also characterized by higher fiber intakes lead to a 59% reduction in high blood pressure risk.

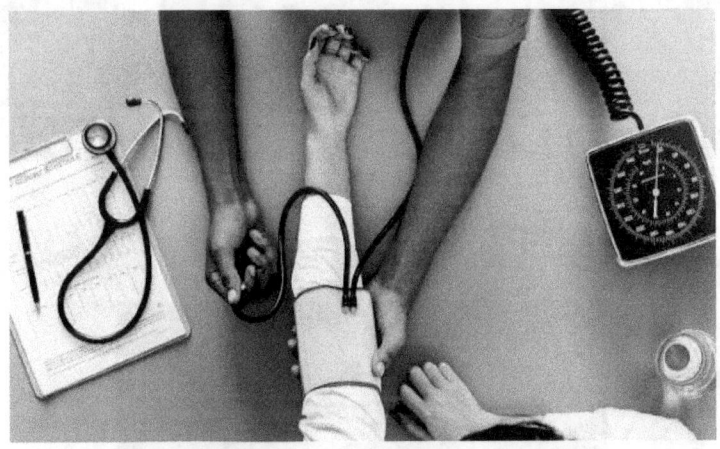

9. Healthy Bones

Osteoporosis is a huge issue, especially for women after menopause. Improving bone health is an important component of treating and preventing osteoporosis. Protein represents key nutrients for bone health. Protein is crucial for the body's ability to absorb calcium and grow bones strong. People who eat more protein tend to have a lower risk of osteoporosis and fractures and maintain better bone mass as they age.

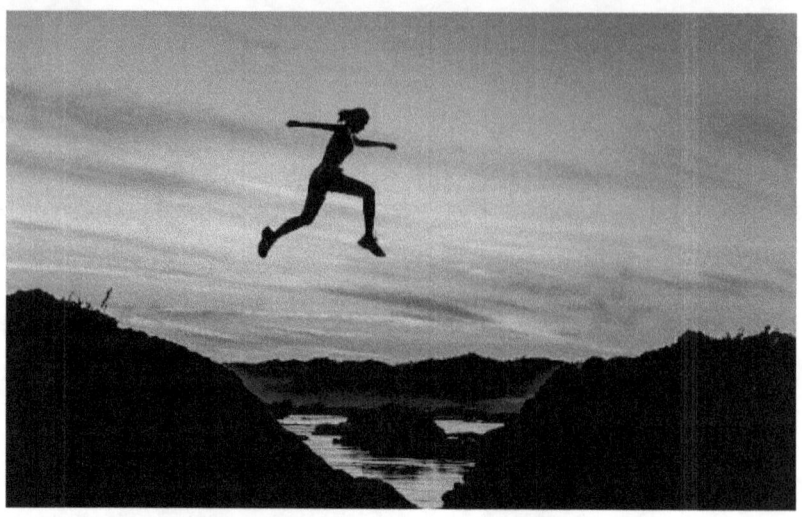

10. Healthy Hair

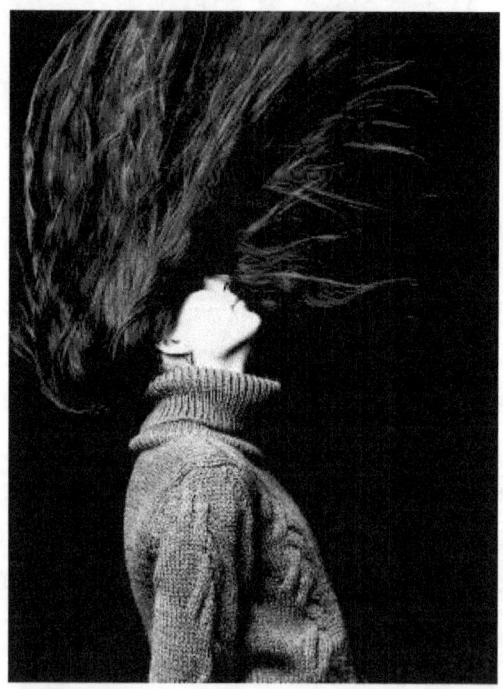

Eating enough protein is important for healthy and strong hair. Protein promotes hair growth because hair follicles are made of mostly protein. A protein-rich diet helps the body to produce keratin, which is fundamental to the hair structure. When keratin weakens, hair strands become dry and brittle. One should eat a high protein and iron-rich diet to prevent hair loss.

Read 10 Most Important Nutrients for Hair Health in the book Secret of Healthy Hair.

Conclusion

Protein is the basic requirement of repairing the body, making enzymes, hormones, and other body chemicals. Increase your protein intake for a healthy life, but remember anything in excess is harmful to health. Eating protein in excess can be harmful to people suffering from kidney disease. Just because protein helps in rapid weight loss, it is never advised to replace carbs and fats with protein in your diet completely. When too much protein is fermented in your stomach, or you are low in digestive acids and enzymes, excess protein can cause bloating, gas, stomach cramps, and diarrhea.

CHAPTER 4

10 High Protein Sources for Vegetarians

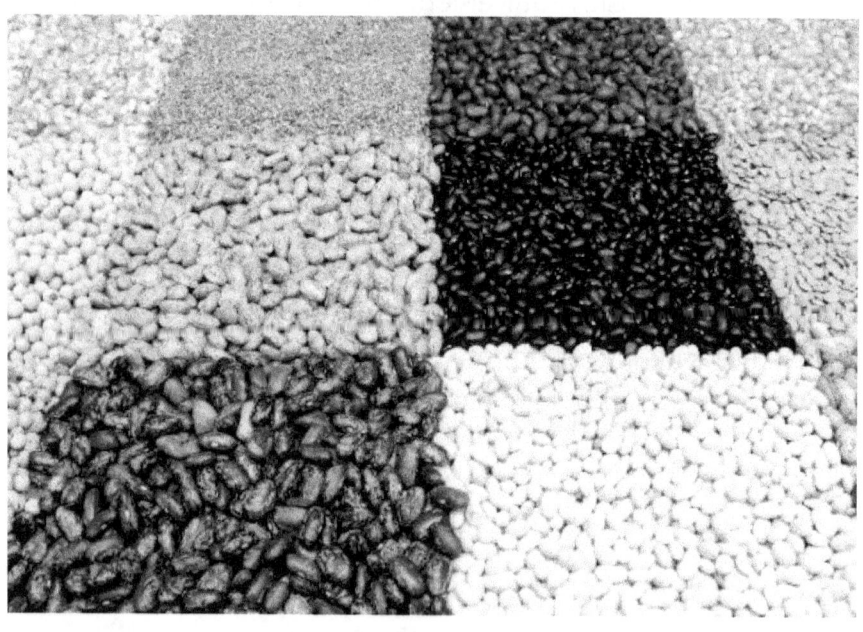

Protein is the building blocks of body tissue such as muscle, hair, bones, nails. Protein deficiency is a very common concern in vegetarian diets. However, animal protein is associated with many degenerative diseases, while vegetable protein isn't.

Sufficient protein intake is a must for all human beings despite age or gender as higher-protein diets boost muscle mass, faster recovery from injury, healthy skin, and weight loss.

Below are the 10 high protein sources for vegetarians:

1. Whey of Cottage Cheese

The liquid portion of the cottage cheese making process is called whey. Whey is a great source of protein for vegetarians. Whey protein helps increase fat loss while providing protein and amino acids, which serve as building blocks for increased muscle growth. You can make cottage cheese by adding 2 tablespoons of lemon juice to 200 ml boiling milk. The acidity of lemon juice will coagulate the milk. Separate the solid and liquid portions. The solid part is the cottage cheese, and the remaining liquid is your whey.

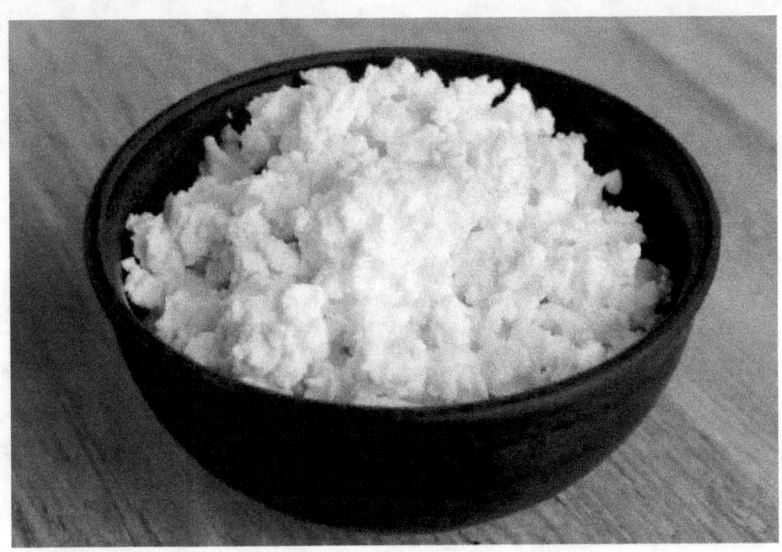

2. Peanuts

Peanuts have more protein than other nuts and are loaded with healthful nutrients, such as antioxidants, fiber, iron, and magnesium. Fats in peanuts are healthful fats, which can help lower bad LDL cholesterol and improve heart health.

100 g of peanuts contain 26 g of protein.

Peanuts recipes: Sabudana Khichdi, Crunchy Peanut Chocolate Bars, Roasted Spicy Peanuts.

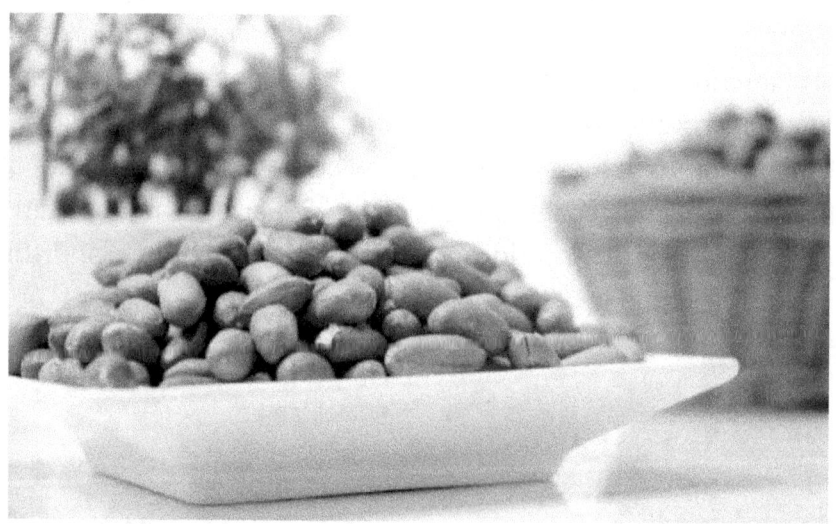

3. Kidney Beans

Kidney beans are low in fats and an excellent source of protein. They are also a good source of fiber, vitamins, and minerals. Kidney beans contain all nine amino acids. They are a good source of lysine, an amino acid usually lacking in other plant-based protein sources, such as grains.

100 g of kidney beans contain 24 g of protein.

Kidney Beans recipes: Mexican Bean Soup, Rajma (Kidney Bean Curry), Vegetarian chili tacos.

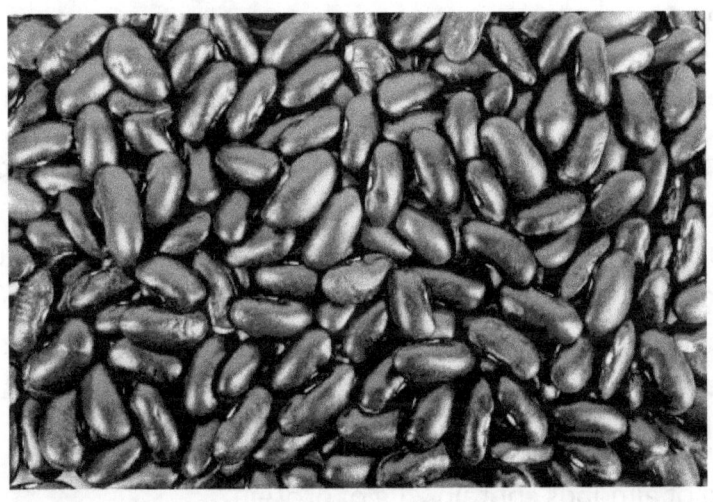

4. Oats

Oats contain more protein than most grains. Oat protein is almost equivalent to soy protein quality, which is equal to meat, milk, and egg protein as per WHO. Oats are one of the easy ways to add protein to your diet.

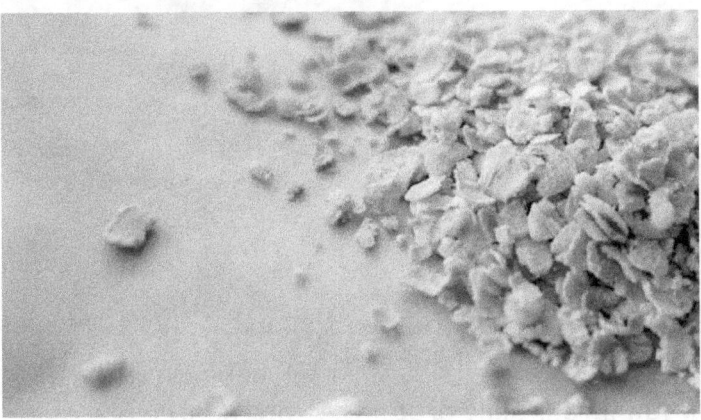

100 g of the hull-less oat kernels contain 12-24 g of protein, the

highest among cereals.

Oats recipes: Vegetable Oats Cutlets, Oatmeal Cookies, Oats Upma.

5. Almonds

Almonds are an excellent source of protein. These are also rich in fiber and vitamin E, which is excellent for the skin. One should eat at least 10 almonds every day, not only for protein but also for its other health benefits. Eat overnight soaked almonds because soaking reduces the number of tannins and acids present in the almond skin, which can inhibit nutrient uptake by the body.

100 g of almonds contain 21 g of protein.

Almonds recipes: Almond Cake, Dry Fruits Milk Shake, Almond Cookies.

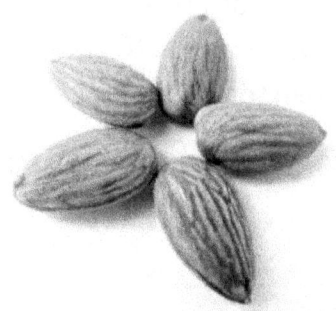

6. Chickpeas

Chickpeas are a great source of protein. There are plenty of chickpeas recipes available that can satisfy your taste bud as well as fulfill your daily protein requirement.

100 g of chickpeas contain 19 g of protein.

Chickpeas recipes: Hummus spread, Falafel, and Indian Chana masala.

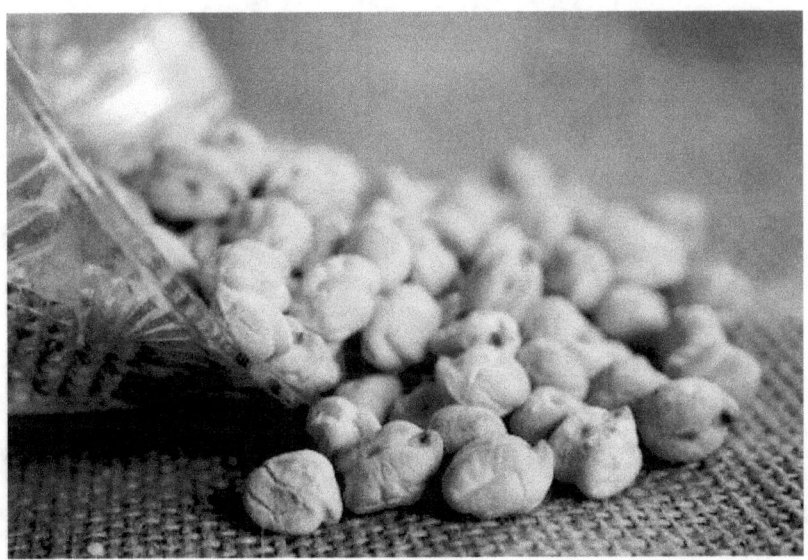

7. Amaranth

Amaranth is a protein powerhouse. Amaranth is high in lysine and protein. Lysine is an amino acid found in low quantities in other grains. Amaranth grain is free from gluten, which makes it a viable grain for people with gluten intolerance. Amaranth is rich in fiber and a good source of manganese, magnesium, vitamin B6, phosphorus, and iron.

100 g of amaranth contains 14 g of protein.

Amaranth recipes: Amaranth and Almond Ladoo, Amaranth cutlets, Amaranth Flour and Raisin Cookies.

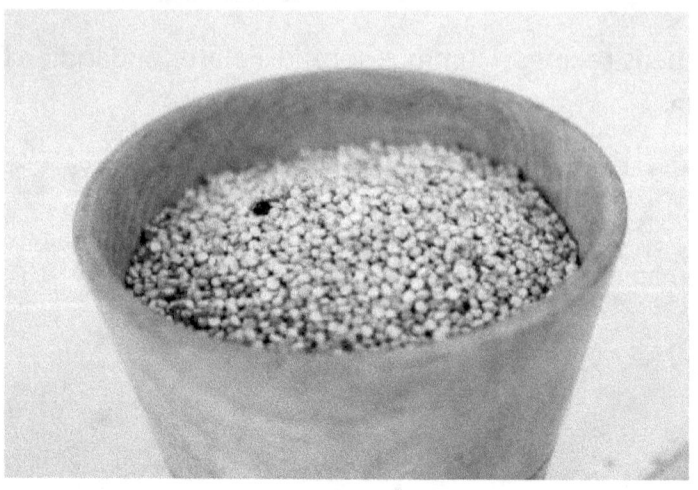

Learn about 10 Worst Foods You Should Avoid for Healthy Hair in the book Secret of Healthy Hair.

8. Greek Yogurt

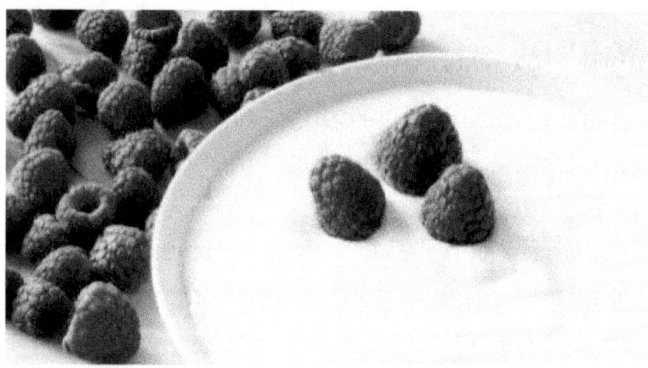

Greek yogurt has more protein than the regular one because Greek yogurt is strained three times, so most whey is removed. It also has lesser carbohydrates than regular yogurt since some of the whey is removed. Because Greek yogurt is more concentrated, it has more protein than regular yogurt.

100 g of Greek yogurt contains 10 g of protein.

Greek Yogurt recipes: Greek Yogurt Pancakes, Salad with Greek Yogurt Dressing, Pasta in Greek Yogurt Sauce.

9. Tofu

Tofu is also known as bean curd. Like cottage cheese, tofu is prepared by coagulating soy milk and pressing the resulting curd into solid white blocks. Tofu is the richest source of protein as it contains all nine essential amino acids. It is also a valuable source of iron, calcium, copper, zinc, vitamin B1, phosphorous, manganese, and selenium.

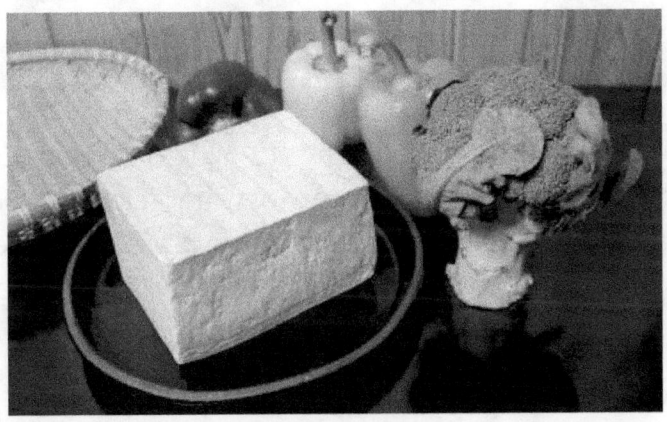

100 g of tofu contains 8 g of protein.

Tofu recipes: Tofu Nuggets, Asian Garlic Tofu, Tofu Manchurian, Chili Tofu.

10. Green Peas

Peas are a complete protein because all nine essential amino acids are present in them. Along with protein, peas have a high level of vitamin K. Additionally peas are a good source of dietary fiber, vitamin A, vitamin C, iron, folate, thiamin, and manganese.

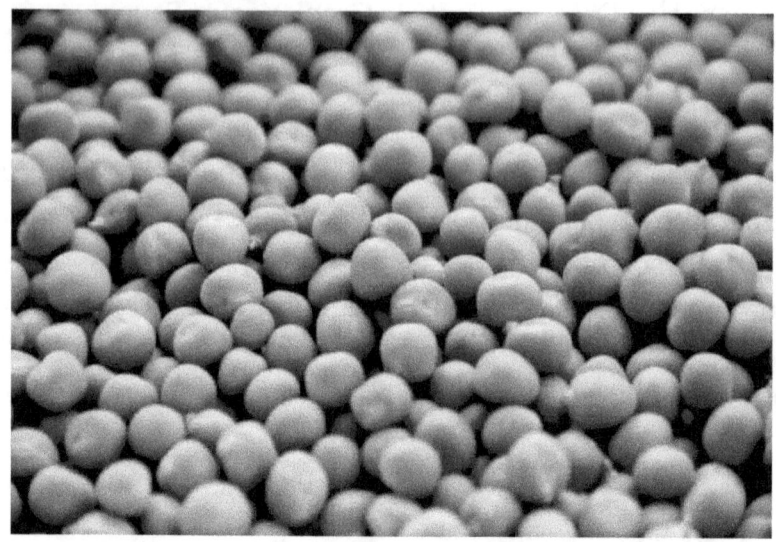

Both fresh and dried green peas are high in protein. You can soak the dried green peas in plenty of water overnight or for 6-8 hours. Drain the water. Place peas in a pressure cooker with 2 cups of water. Pressure cook for 1 whistle. Now it is ready to use in your recipes.

100 g of Peas contain 6 g of protein.

Green Peas recipes: Green Peas Cutlet, Peas Fried Rice, Peas, and Mint Soup.

My Thoughts

Protein is the building block of bones, muscles, skin, and nails. Our body requires protein for repairing and making enzymes, hormones, and other chemicals of the body. Insufficient protein intake in vegetarians is not uncommon. The above-listed protein-rich foods are readily available in the market, and anyone can easily include these in their diet.

CHAPTER 5

10 Reasons Why Fat is Not the Enemy. The Truth About Fats!

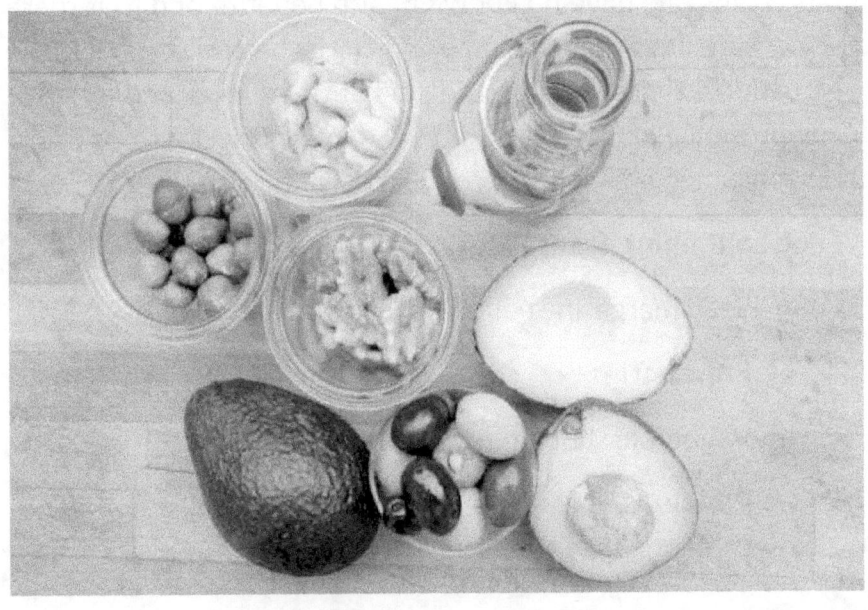

Did you know that the human brain is made up of nearly 60% fat? Fats are not something we should run from; our body needs a certain amount of fat to function at its best. Not all fats are bad, not all fats are good. Let's just quickly see which type of fat is our friend and which one is our enemy.

Types of Fats:

Trans Fats

Trans fats are the *worst* type of dietary fat. The hydrogenation process is used to turn healthy oils into solids to prevent them from becoming rancid, and a byproduct of this process is Trans fats. Trans fats have no known health benefits, and that there is no safe level of consumption. It is better to check the Nutritional Facts label on the packet of your packed food for any presence of trans fat. For every 2% of calories from trans-fat consumed daily, the risk of heart disease rises by 23%.

Food containing Trans Fat:

- Solid margarine
- French fries
- Vegetable shortening
- Pastries
- Cookies

Saturated Fats

They are solid at room temperature. A diet rich in saturated fats can increase total cholesterol, particularly harmful LDL cholesterol, that may cause blockages in arteries in the heart or elsewhere in the body. Saturated fat should be consumed in moderation, and it is recommended to limit the consumption of saturated fat to less than 10% calories a day.

Common sources of saturated fat:

- Whole milk
- Cheese
- Red meat
- Coconut oil
- Many commercially prepared baked goods

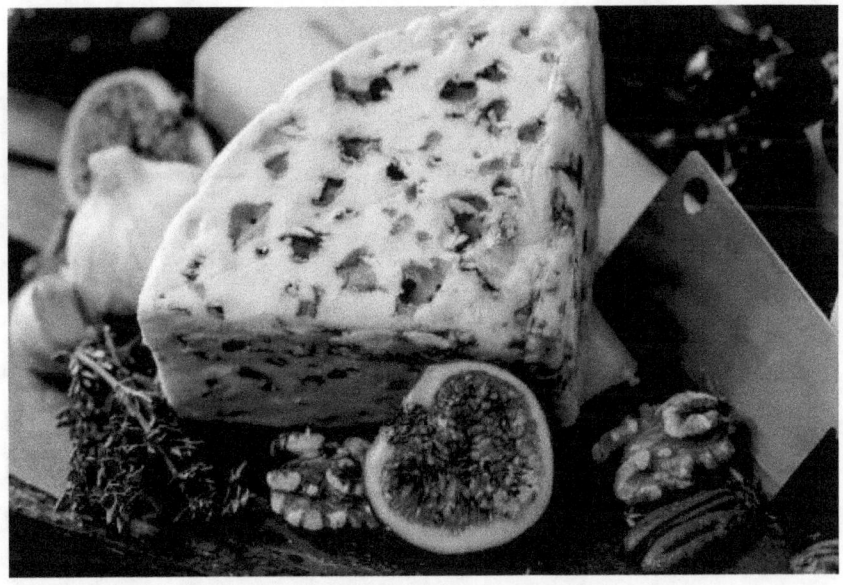

Unsaturated Fats

Monounsaturated and Polyunsaturated Fats

Monounsaturated and Polyunsaturated fats are healthy fats. They are liquid at room temperature and found in vegetables, nuts, and seeds. Polyunsaturated fats build cell membranes and the covering of nerves. They play an important role in blood clotting, muscle movement, and inflammation.

Good sources of monounsaturated fats are

- Extra virgin olive oil
- Sunflower oil
- Peanut oil
- Canola oil
- High-oleic safflower oil
- Avocado
- Nuts

Omega-3 fatty acids and omega-6 fatty acids are examples of polyunsaturated fats. Replacing saturated fats and refined carbohydrates with polyunsaturated fats can reduce harmful LDL cholesterol and improves the cholesterol profile. It also lowers triglycerides.

Good sources of omega-3 fatty acids include

- Flax seeds
- Chia seeds

- kidney beans
- Soybeans
- Walnut

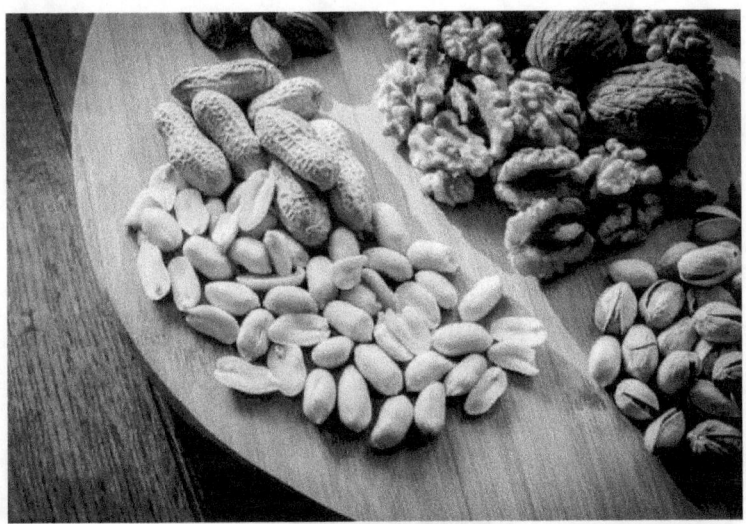

Omega-6 fatty acids have been linked to protection against heart disease.

Good sources of omega-6 fatty acids include

- Corn oil
- Sunflower oil
- Safflower oil
- Soybean oil
- Walnut

Below are the 10 reasons why fat is not the enemy:

1. Fat is Essential to Brain Health

Fat is essential to brain health. The brain is made of 60% fats, out of which a large chunk is docosahexaenoic acid (DHA) or Omega 3 fat.

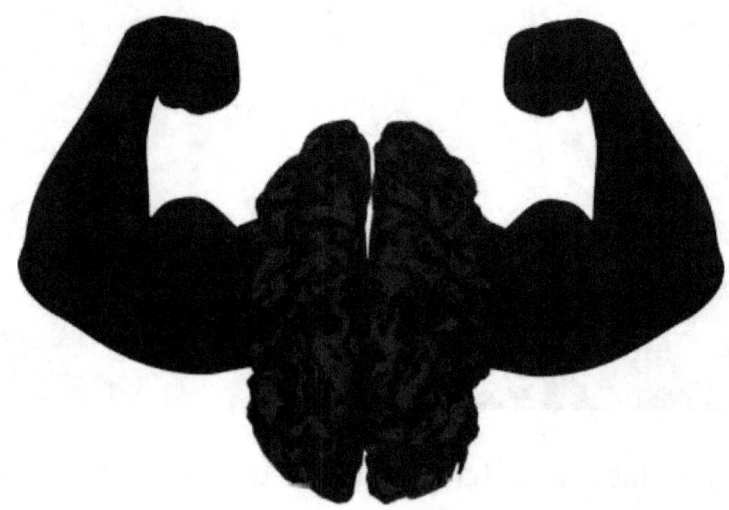

Essential fat-soluble vitamins such as A, D, E, and K are not water-soluble and require fat to get transported and absorbed in the body. These fat-soluble vitamins are crucial for brain health and many of our vital organs.

Vitamin D decreases susceptibility to Alzheimer's, Parkinson's, depression, and other brain disorders, and omega-3 is said to sharpen cognitive function and improve mood.

2. Fat for Better Skin

Fat makes up the bulk of the cellular membrane, and our skin is made up of a large number of cells. Without the proper consumption of fat, skin can become dry and chapped, which can also open up pathways for infection to enter our body.

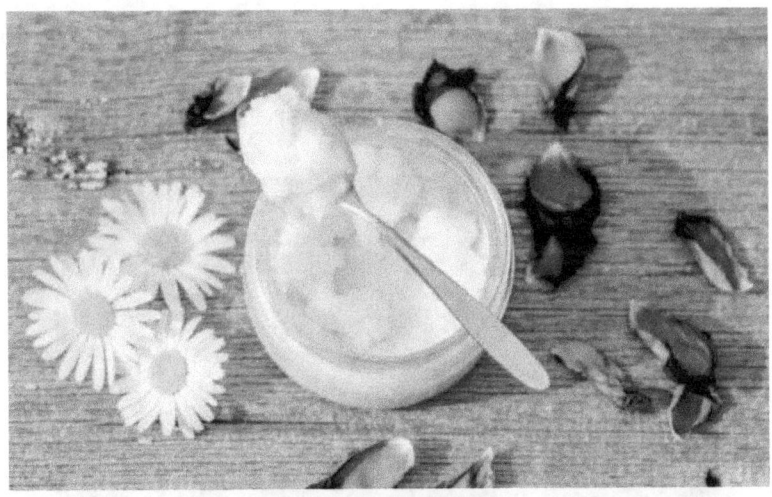

3. Fat Boosts Immune System

Fats are required for a healthy immune system. Saturated fats play an important role here, as adequate amounts will help the immune system recognize and then destroy foreign invaders.

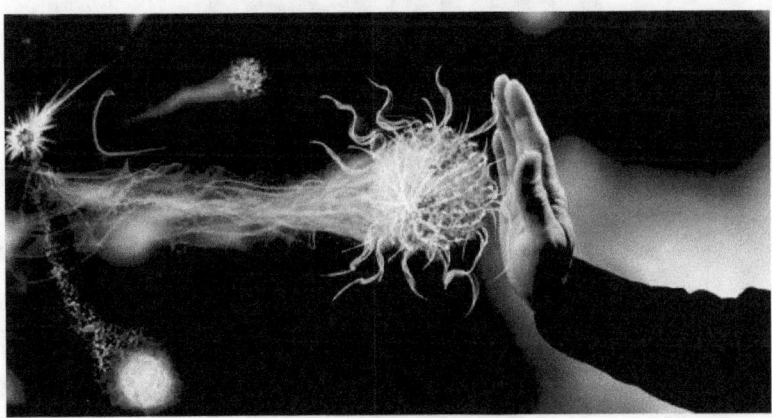

*Learn What are the Power Foods to Boost Your Immunity in the book Eat to Prevent and Controls Disease.

4. Fat Keeps Our Lungs Working Properly

Lungs are coated with a thin layer that is made up of 100% saturated fat. Fats are needed to protect this protective layer; Otherwise, it may result in breathing problems.

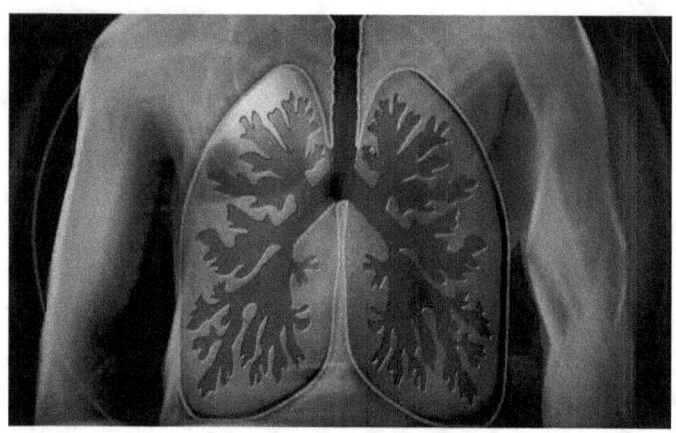

5. Fat is Good for Heart

Unsaturated fats are healthy for your heart because they help lower blood pressure and slows the build-up of plaque in arteries by reducing triglycerides, a type of fat in your blood. Switching from saturated fats to polyunsaturated or monounsaturated fats can lower heart disease risk by up to 25%.

6. Fat Can Help You Lose Weight (Yes, you read it right)

Hungry cells cause weight gain. When you limit your calorie intake, your body goes into starvation mode, holding onto calories and storing fat.

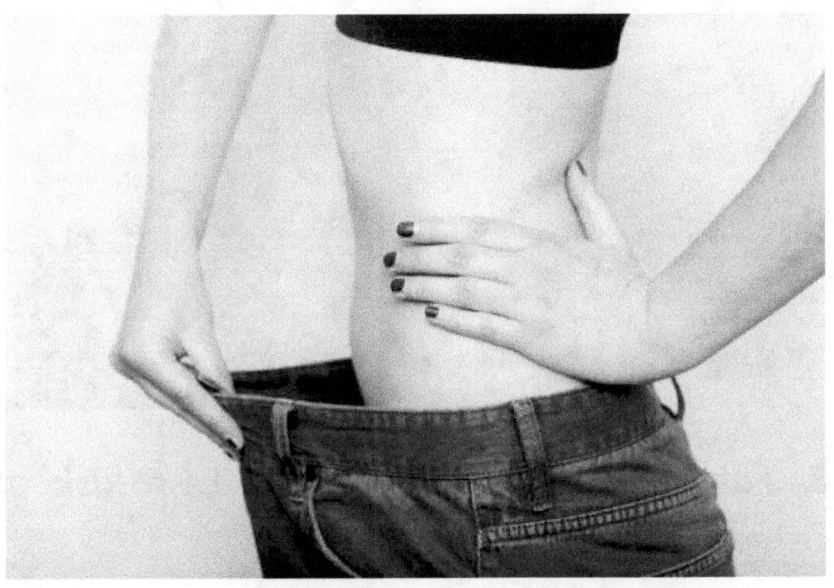

When you fuel your body with the right foods and enough healthy fats, your metabolism keeps running, and you are better at losing weight.

7. Fat for Proper Insulin Release

Saturated fats found in coconut oil help support proper nerve signaling by acting on signaling messengers. These messengers affect metabolism, as well as control the proper release of insulin.

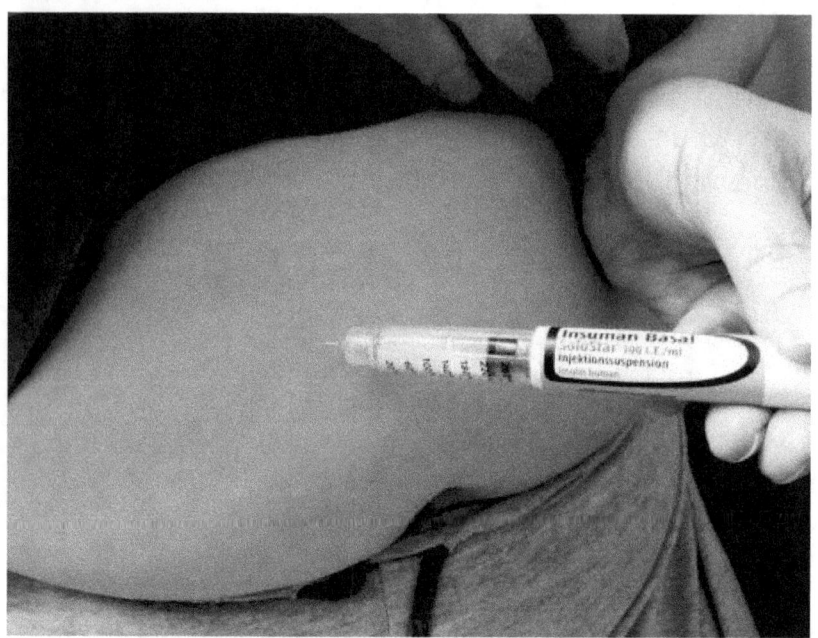

8. Fat for Stronger Bones and Less Risk of Osteoporosis

The important bone-building vitamins – Vitamin A, D, E, and K are only fat-soluble, which means they are transported and absorbed using dietary fats. Fat is required for the metabolism of calcium.

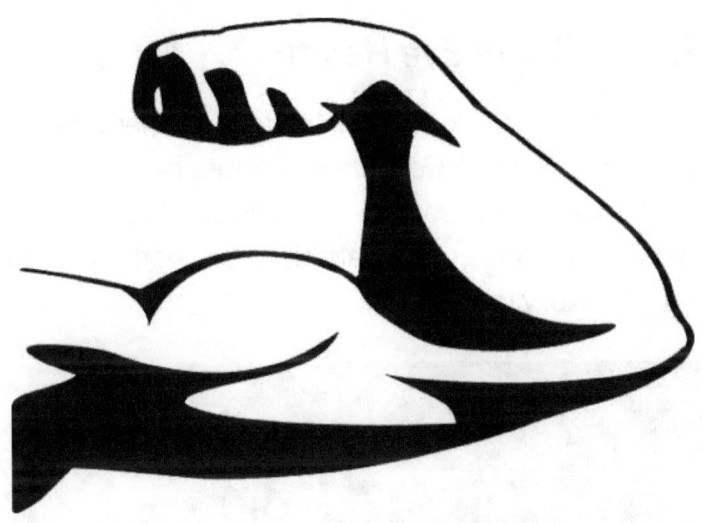

9. Fat for Better Reproductive Health

Fats are the building blocks for healthy cell membranes and are important for hormonal health. Sex hormones – testosterone, estrogen, progesterone – are all made of cholesterol. Cutting way back on dietary fats can increase your risk of hormonal problems like hypothyroidism, menstrual irregularities, and low testosterone levels for men.

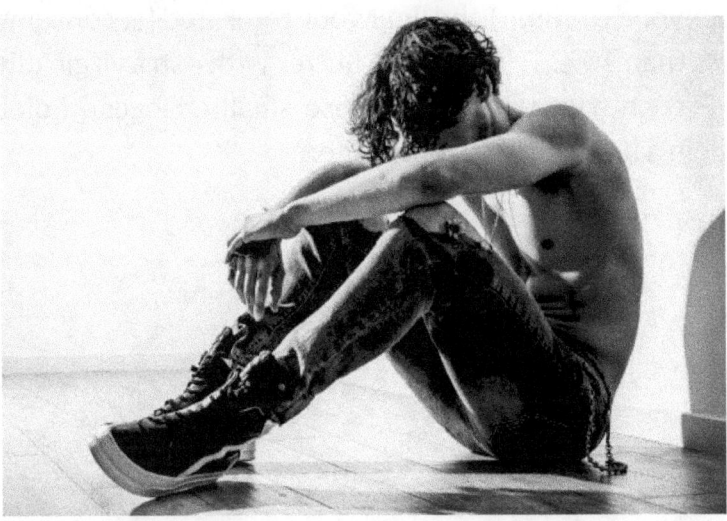

10. Fat for Better Eye Health

In dry eye disease, lack of tears leads to dryness, discomfort, and occasional blurry vision. Omega-3 fats help produce more tears and may benefit people with this condition. In addition, omega-3 fats help prevent diabetic retinopathy due to their anti-inflammatory properties.

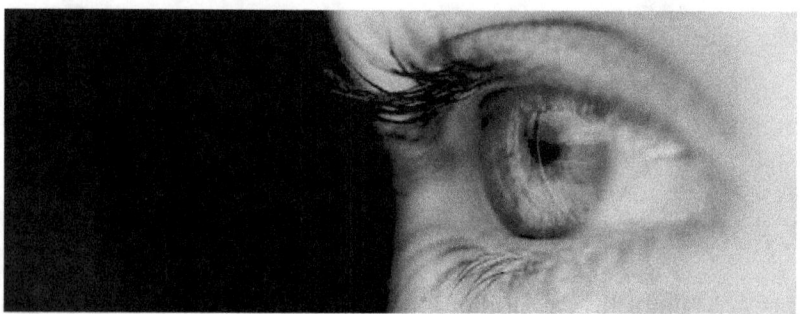

Conclusion

No doubt not all fats are good for health, but at the same time, certain types of fats are essential for our health. Try to eat monounsaturated and polyunsaturated fats as much as you can (not beyond the limit) and limit your saturated fat consumption to less than 10%. Try replacing butter with extra virgin olive oil and French fries with nuts. These small changes in diet will result in a healthier and longer life.

CHAPTER 6

Top 10 Healthy Fat Foods You Should Eat

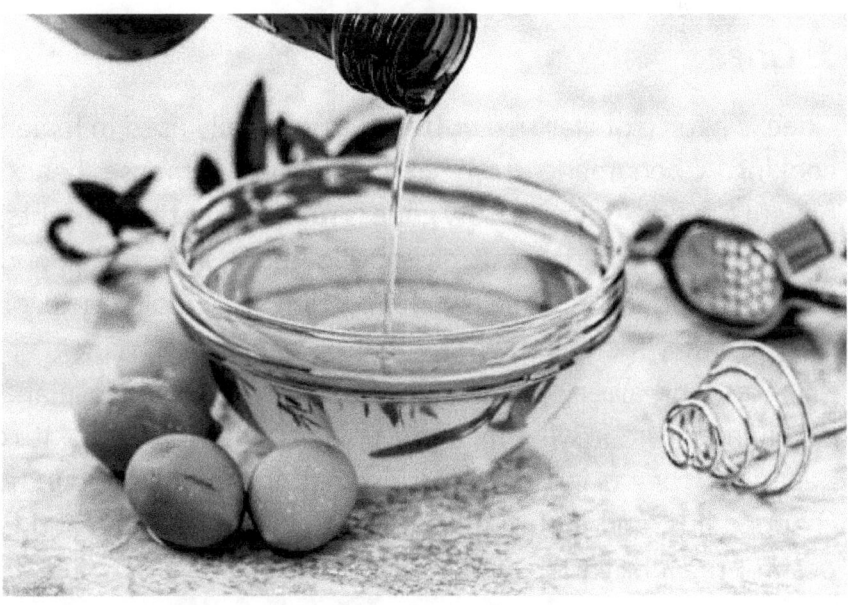

From decades fat is associated with weight gain, heart diseases, and many more. But now is the time you understand all types of fats are not the devil. If you avoid fats but have no control over sugar, processed and refined carbs consumption, it is more dangerous to your health. Fat not only stores energy but insulates and protects vital organs. In fact, healthy fats boost your heart health, improve cholesterol levels and enhance your beauty by making your skin glowing and hair shiny.

Focus more on foods rich in unsaturated fats (monounsaturated and polyunsaturated) but don't 100% avoid saturated fats.

Below I have listed the top 10 healthy fat sources you should eat for health and nutritional benefits.

1. Ghee

Ghee is a form of clarified butter. It is generally used in Indian cooking. Ghee made from cow milk has immense health benefits as per Ayurved. Cow ghee is full of essential nutrients, fatty acids, antioxidants. It has antibacterial, anti-fungal, and antiviral properties. Ghee is rich in conjugated linoleic acid, or CLA, a fatty acid known to protect against carcinogens, diabetes, and artery plaque. It is known as a brain tonic and excellent for improving memory power and intelligence. It is beneficial for curing thyroid dysfunction. It heals wounds, chapped lips, and mouth ulcers. It also cures insomnia and is best for the lubrication of joints.

Ghee has a high smoke point which means ghee doesn't go rancid even at high temperature and retains all the important nutrients that provide all the incredible ghee benefits. Ghee is a rich source of vitamin A, vitamin E, and vitamin K, keeping your skin glowing and maintaining healthy vision. Vitamin K found in ghee helps prevent calcium deposits in the arteries that can obstruct blood flow and lead to blockages. Ghee should consume in moderation if you don't want to put on weight. 1 tablespoon (15g) of ghee in a day is enough to ripe all the health benefits of ghee.

2. Extra Virgin Olive Oil

Extra virgin olive oil is one of the world's healthiest oils. Eating about 2 tablespoons of extra virgin olive oil every day may reduce the risk of coronary heart disease due to the presence of monounsaturated fats in olive oil. Extra virgin olive oil is loaded with powerful antioxidants that inhibit oxidation and prevent the formation of free radicals in the body, which reduce the risk of chronic diseases and cancer.

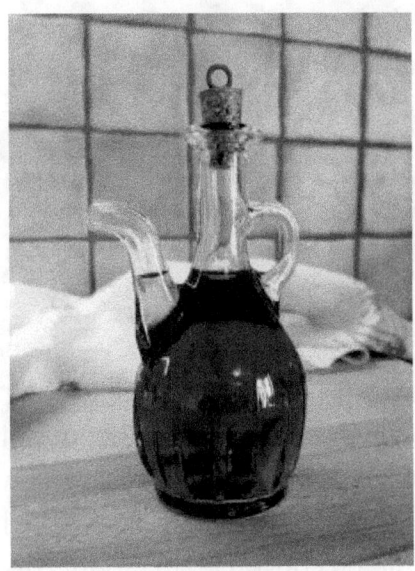

Do not use extra virgin olive oil for cooking at high temperatures, such as deep-frying, as it oxidizes quicker than other oils.

3. Coconut & Coconut Oil

Lauric acid is why coconut is considered healthy, even though it contains almost 89% of saturated fats. Lauric acid, a 12-carbon atom chain, is a saturated fatty acid found in coconut with antibacterial, antiviral, and antimicrobial properties that prevent infections. Coconut oil is good for your skin and hair.

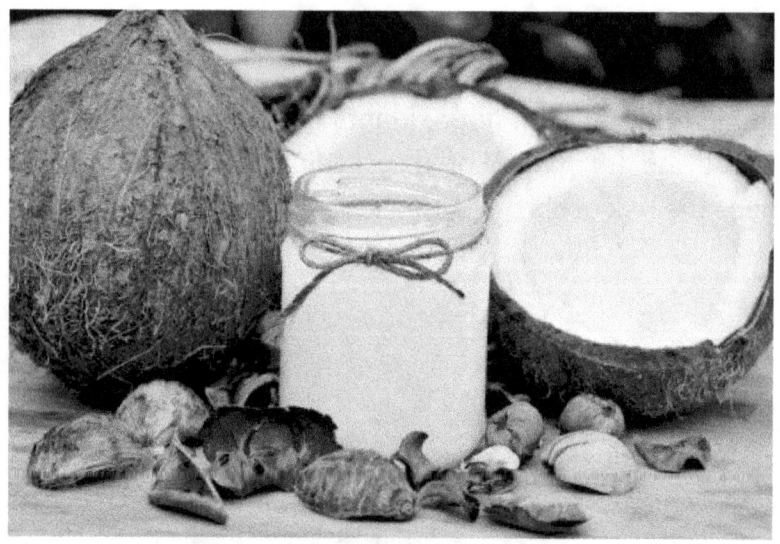

Coconut oil has anti-inflammatory properties due to antioxidants present in it, potentially helping to reduce arthritis symptoms. Saturated fat in coconut oil increases HDL levels (good cholesterol) and promotes heart health, but at the same time, it increases LDL levels (bad cholesterol) too; therefore, it should be consumed in moderation.

Read Top 10 Foods that Prevent Hair Loss and Promote Hair Growth in the book Secret of Healthy Hair.

4. Avocado

Avocado is loaded with vitamin B complex, vitamin K, vitamin C, and vitamin E. It is also rich in phytosterols and carotenoids such as lutein and zeaxanthin. These carotenoids are converted into vitamin A in the body and protect the eyes from diseases by absorbing harmful blue light entering the eyes. Vitamin K in avocado can support bone health by increasing calcium absorption.

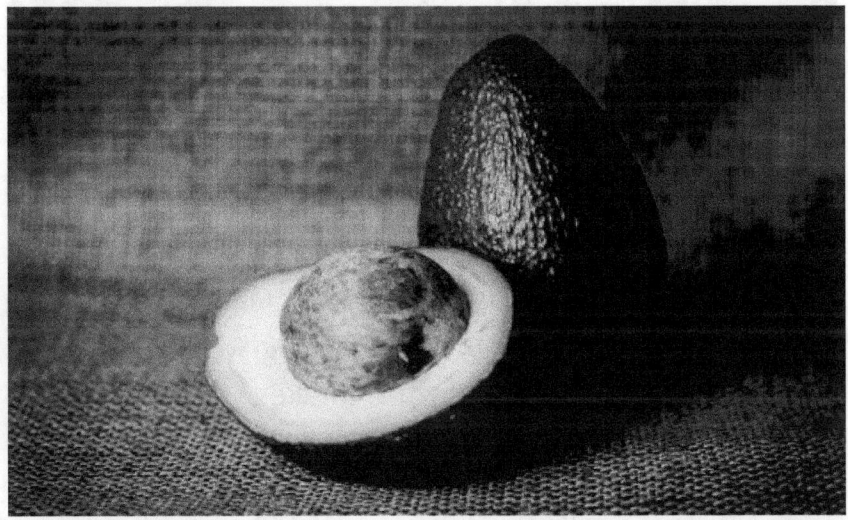

Dietary fiber in avocado improves digestion. About 75% of an avocado's calories come from fat, mostly monounsaturated fats MUFAs (about 65%) like oleic acid and linoleic acid. These monounsaturated fats are strongly associated with reduced risks of developing diabetes, heart disease, and high blood pressure.

5. Flaxseeds

Flaxseeds are high in unsaturated omega-3 fatty acids: alpha-linolenic acid (ALA), which protects against heart disease by improving blood pressure. Only 1-2 tablespoons of Flaxseeds are enough to reap the benefits.

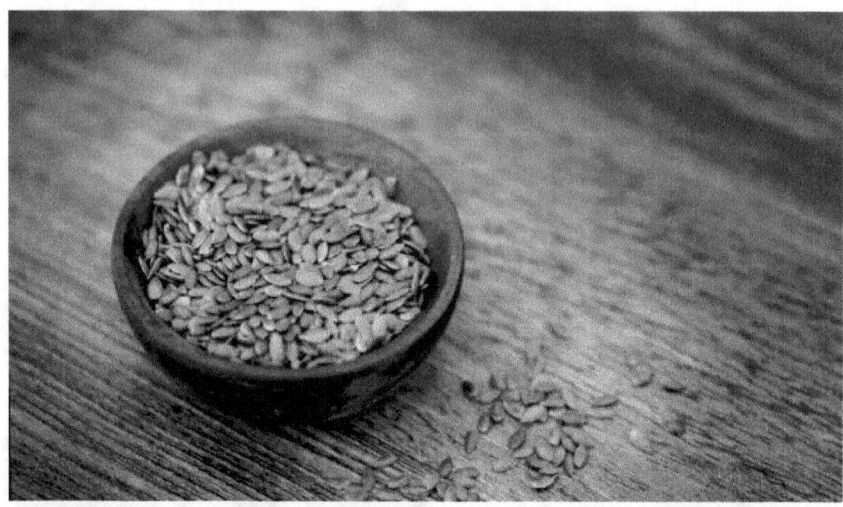

Flaxseed contains both soluble and insoluble fiber that leaves you feeling full for a long time, reducing weight as well as lowering cholesterol levels. Regular intake of flaxseeds is good for your skin and heart. Flaxseeds contain other nutrients such as protein, magnesium, calcium, phosphorus, omega-3, and lignin. Lignans in flaxseed have antioxidant and estrogen properties that prevent cancer.

6. Black Sesame Seeds

Black sesame seeds are high in unsaturated fatty acids while low in saturated fatty acids. Black sesame is considered one of the best anti-aging foods according to traditional Chinese medicine. Sesame seeds are high in calcium, magnesium, and copper, which are bone-forming minerals.

The oleic acid and linoleic acid in black sesame seeds promote skin softening and cell regeneration, improving skin health. The higher iron content of black sesame seeds helps in preventing iron-deficiency anemia.

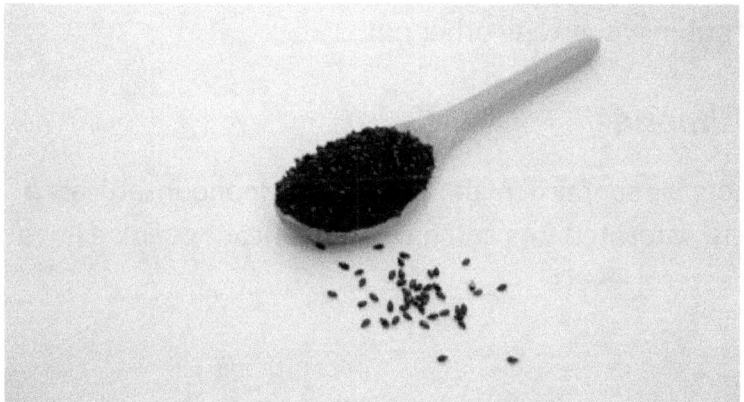

7. Walnuts

Unlike most nuts, walnuts are high in polyunsaturated fatty acids - omega-3 fats, especially alpha-linolenic acid (ALA), linoleic acid, and oleic acid, which protects against heart disease.

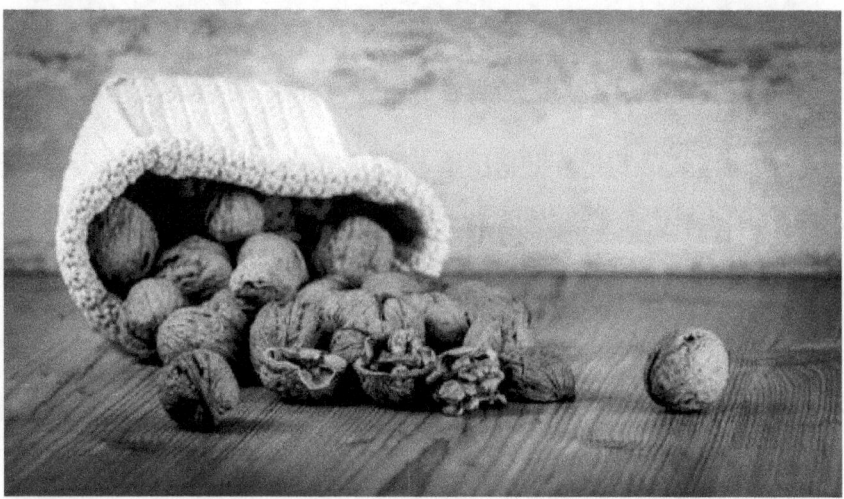

Eat walnuts for better brain function and better memory. Walnuts may help lower blood pressure. The anti-inflammatory property of walnut reduces the risk of breast and prostate cancers. Antioxidants in walnut are of higher quality and potency than any other nut.

8. Almonds

Almonds contain high levels of monounsaturated and polyunsaturated fats and have a significant positive impact on cholesterol levels.

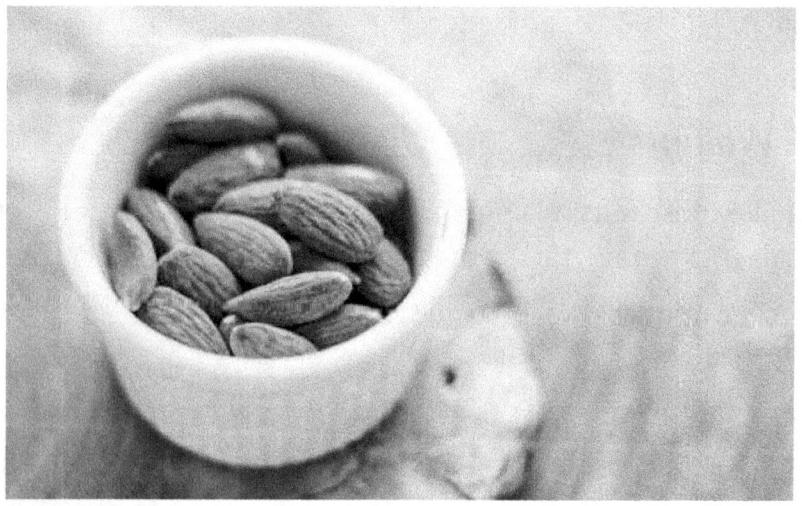

The protein and fiber content of almonds make them the best option for snack because a handful of almonds can satisfy you for at least a few hours, increasing your chances of losing weight successfully. Biotin (also known as vitamin H) in almonds improves hair health. Almonds are rich in vitamin E and antioxidants, which improve skin health.

9. Dark Chocolate

Dark chocolate is rich in flavanols, a powerful antioxidant that can lower blood pressure and allow more blood to flow to the heart, therefore improving heart health. Although half of the dark chocolate fat content is saturated fats, it is a good source of vitamins A, B, and E, iron, calcium, potassium, magnesium.

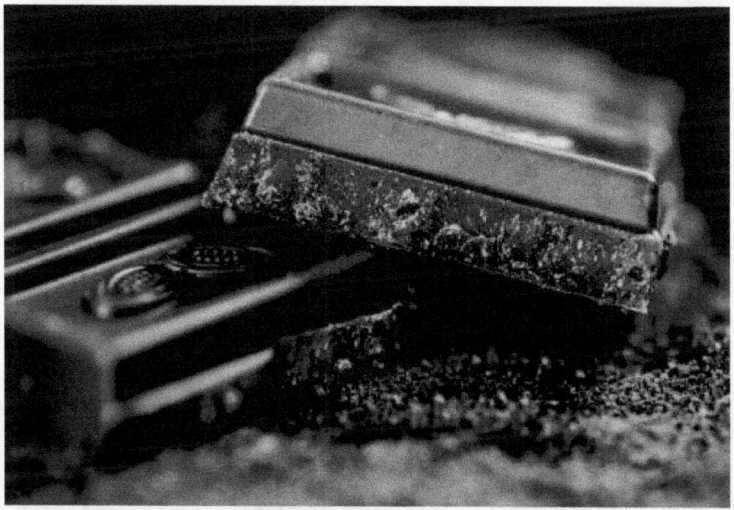

Also, dark chocolate helps improve cognitive performance but make sure you eat chocolate with 70 percent cocoa for the highest flavonoids and avoid milk chocolate, which contains loads of sugar and dairy.

10. Dairy

Cow's milk is good for the bones because it is a rich source of calcium, an essential mineral for healthy bones and teeth. Cow's milk is a good source of potassium, which can reduce blood pressure, and risk of cardiovascular disease.

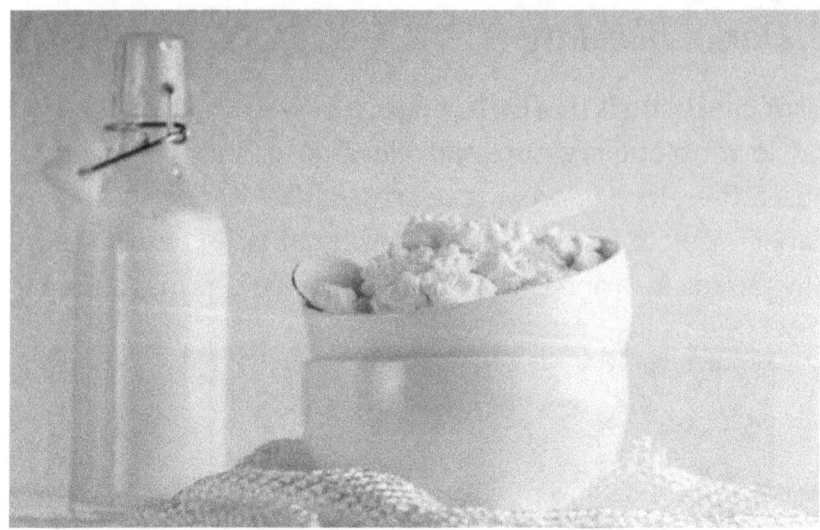

Some available **Cheese** options are healthy as they fulfill the body's calcium and potassium need. Cottage cheese, feta, ricotta are the top healthiest cheese options available.

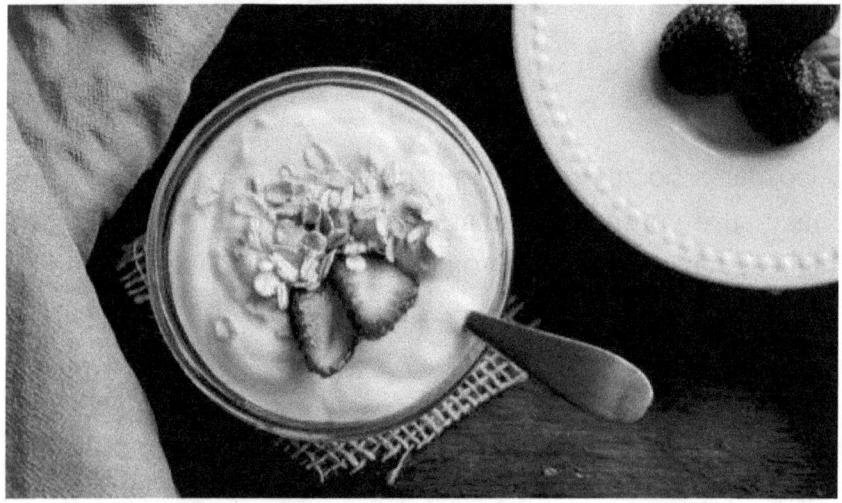

Probiotic yogurt helps keep the intestine healthy and strengthen the digestive tract. Probiotic yogurt increases the good bacteria in your gut to promote better overall health.

Daily intake of probiotic yogurt boosts immunity and reduces cholesterol levels.

Conclusion

Fats are an important dietary requirement. Healthy fats not only provide energy but also protect our vital organs by insulating body organs against shock. Fat-soluble vitamins such as vitamins A, D, E, and K can only be digested and absorbed in conjunction with fats. This proves fats are not the enemy. Start adding healthy fats to your diet from today. Happy eating.

CHAPTER 7

---

10 Reasons You Should Never Give Up Carbohydrates

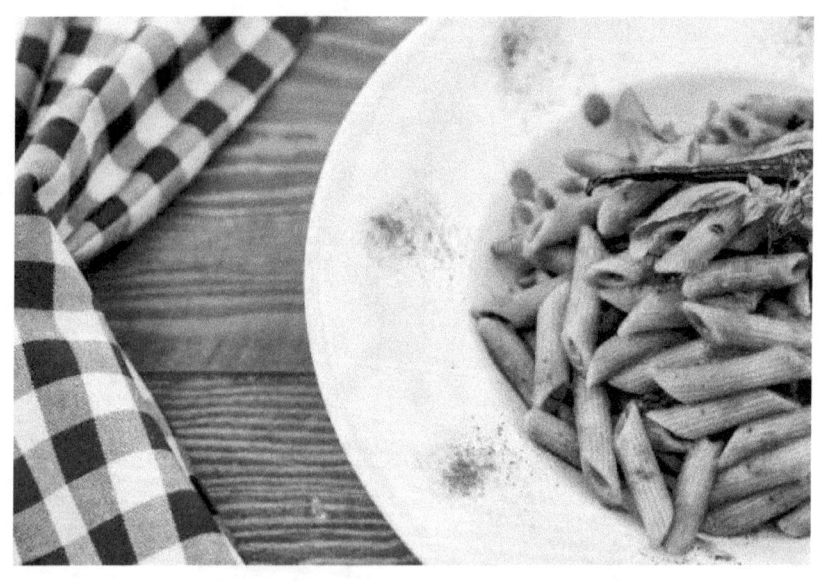

The main function of carbohydrates is to provide the body and brain with energy. Just like your car needs fuel to make it run, your body needs carbohydrates to make it go.

What are Carbohydrates?

Carbohydrates are one of three macronutrients — along with proteins and fats — that your body requires daily. There are three main types of carbohydrates: starches, fiber, and sugars.

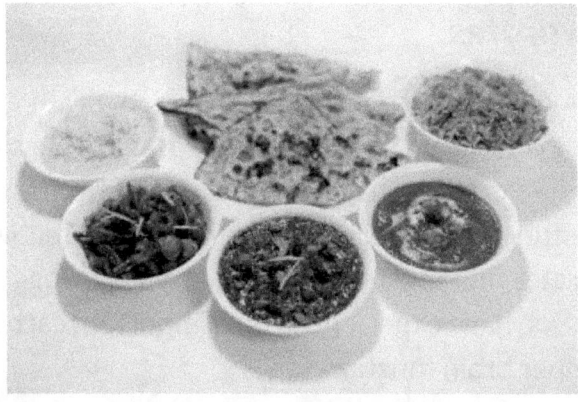

Starches are often referred to as complex carbohydrates. They are found in grains, legumes, and starchy vegetables, like potatoes and corn (*Preferable carbs*).

Sugars are known as simple carbohydrates. There are natural sugars in vegetables, fruits, milk, and honey. Added sugars are found in processed foods, syrups, sugary drinks, and sweets (*Avoidable carbs*).

After you enjoy a meal, the carbohydrates from the food you consumed are broken down into smaller sugar units. These sugar units get absorbed into your bloodstream. Blood sugar is transported through the blood to supply energy to your muscles and other tissues. This is an important process; in fact,

providing energy to the body is the primary role of carbohydrates.

You must get at least 200 to 400 grams of carbs every day. Still not convinced carbs are fine? Then pay attention to these 10 important benefits of eating carbs:

10 reasons you should never give up carbohydrates:

1. Want to Increase Your IQ Level, Eat Carbohydrates

Your body cells require the simple carbohydrate glucose for energy, but your brain particularly needs glucose as an energy source. So, we can say that supplying energy to the brain is an important function of carbs. If you have ever followed a low carbohydrates diet and felt like your brain was foggy for a few days, then you have experienced how important carbohydrates are for proper brain function.

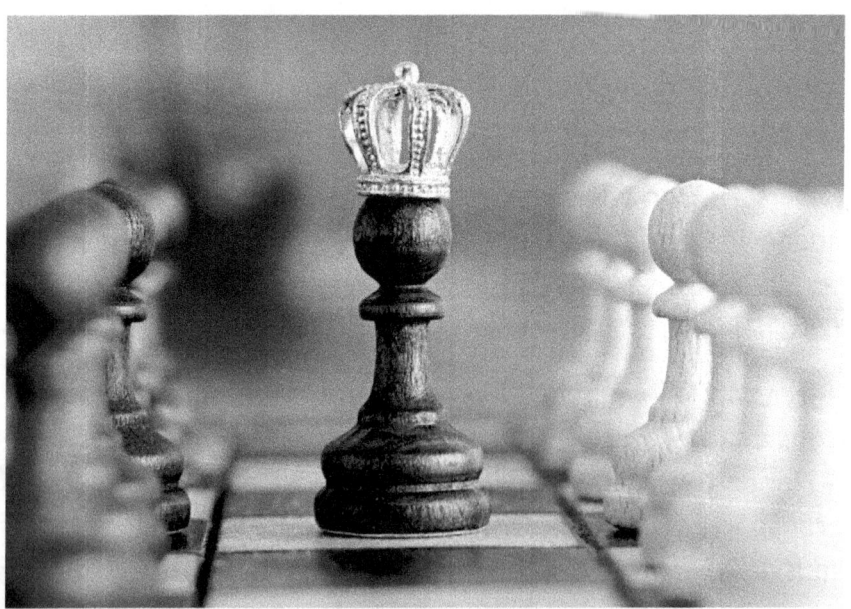

2. Carbohydrates Can Help Boost Your Mood

Carbohydrates promote the production of serotonin, a happy brain chemical. Serotonin is a mood regulator. It keeps you happy and away from depression. In a study, a very low carbohydrate diet was found to increase depression, fatigue, anxiety, and anger than a low-fat, high-carb diet that focuses on whole grains, fruit, and beans.

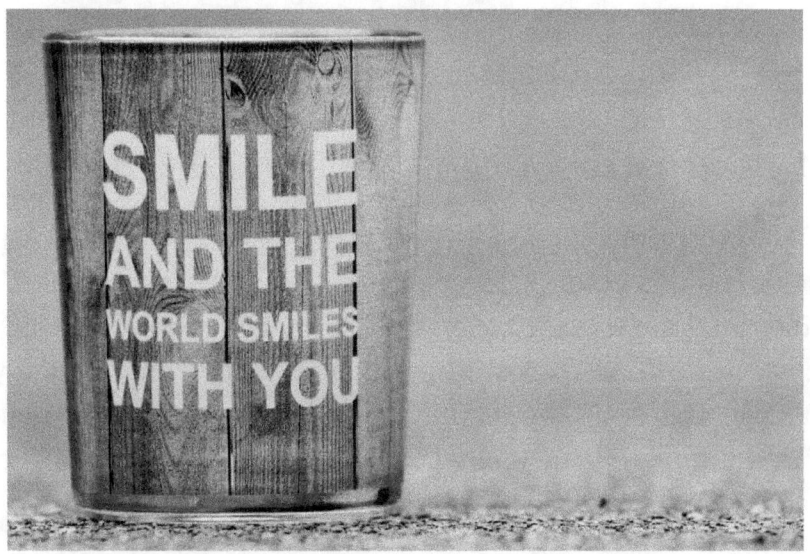

3. Carbohydrates Can Promote Weight Loss

Increasing your soluble fiber intake is an excellent way to promote weight loss. Many carbohydrates contain indigestible dietary fiber, which is a complex carbohydrate that digests more slowly. Soluble fiber dissolves in water and converts into a gel that digests more slowly, making you feel fuller for a longer period. This helps to curb hunger, and you consume fewer calories. As a result, you lose more weight. Make sure you drink enough water with soluble fiber-rich foods to prevent constipation.

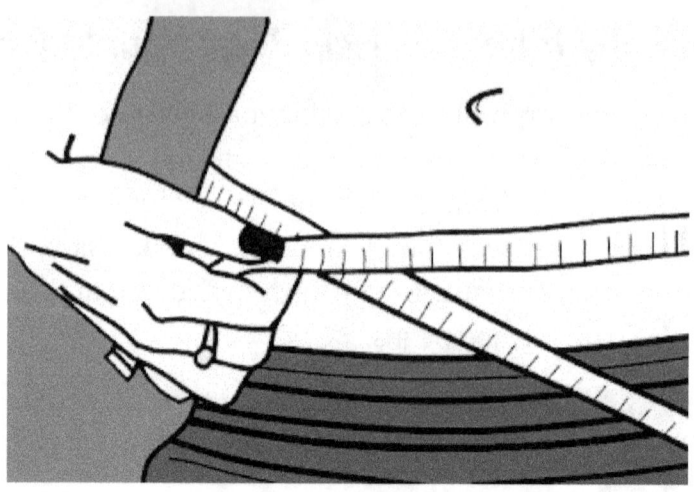

4. Good for Your Heart

Carbohydrates-rich foods like oatmeal and beans contain soluble fiber. Research suggests that increasing your soluble fiber intake by 5 to 10 grams each day could drop your LDL cholesterol (bad cholesterol) levels by 5 percent. Similarly, people who eat more whole grains (brown rice, bulgur, and quinoa) tend to have lower LDL cholesterol levels and higher "good" HDL cholesterol levels.

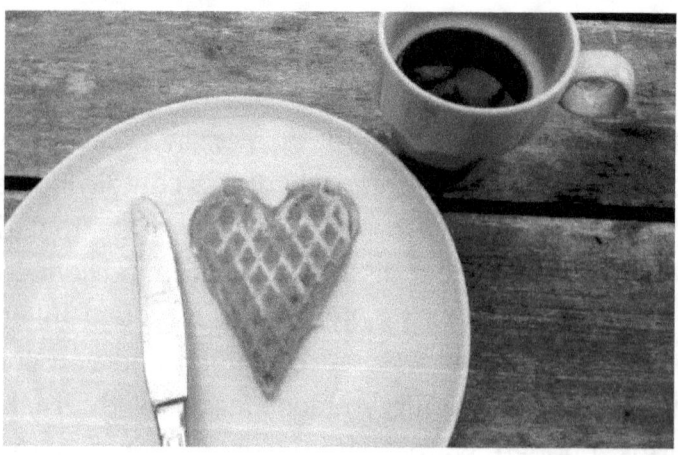

5. Carbohydrates Improve Sleep Pattern

Slow-digested carbohydrate-rich foods increase serotonin release and contribute to restful sleep. Serotonin is not only a mood-enhancing neurotransmitter, in fact, it also helps ensure a comfortable sleep experience. When your diet is low in carbohydrates, your body has a hard time synthesizing serotonin, resulting in insomnia. This is why drinking a glass of warm milk at night is considered good for restful sleep, even though it is not the best carbohydrate option.

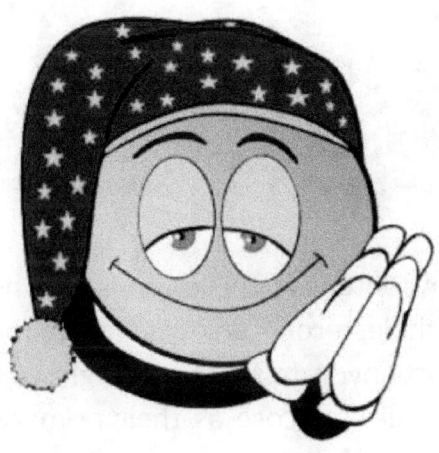

6. Carbohydrates Reduce Cancer Risk

This is a catch-22 and depends a lot on which carbohydrates you opt for. While most people will think of potatoes when considering carbs options, in reality, there are many more options of carbs that might not have crossed your mind. For example, onions, tomatoes, bell peppers, and hundreds of vegetables can all be considered carbohydrates at their core, even though what they bring to the table are vastly different. These are the carbohydrates you should be aiming for. These are loaded with antioxidants and help to combat abnormal cellular growth.

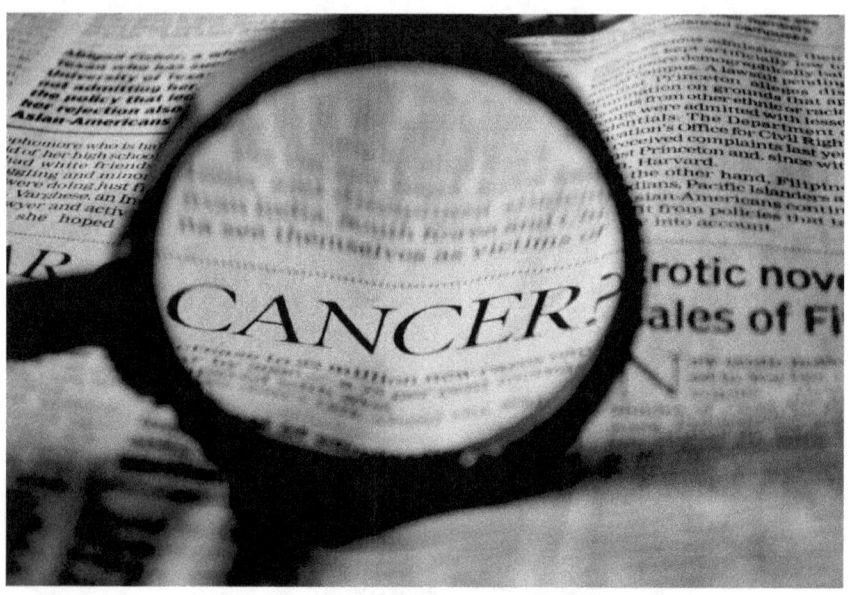

The high fiber content of these foods also helps to promote waste and cholesterol removal from the body. These wholesome carbohydrate foods also fight early-stage cancer, as the cells require glucose as their primary source of fuel. Consuming foods that very slowly convert to glucose can reduce the supply of nutrients to them, and cell death or apoptosis may occur.

7. Carbohydrates Improve Digestion

Getting enough fiber-rich carbohydrates is the key to prevent digestive problems, such as constipation and indigestion. Carbohydrates rich foods contain insoluble fiber, which does not dissolve in water and is left intact during digestion, which is also known as roughage. It pushes other foods through the gastrointestinal tract, speeding up the digestion process. Also, it adds bulk to your stool, making it easier to pass stool. Without sufficient intake of carbohydrates, you may not get enough fiber to keep your digestive system regular.

8. Carbohydrates Improve Blood Pressure

High blood pressure is among the significant risk factors for stroke and heart disease. Therefore, lowering blood pressure is an effective way to reduce the risk of heart disease. Studies have indicated that diets rich in carbohydrates lowers blood pressure in overweight or obese individuals.

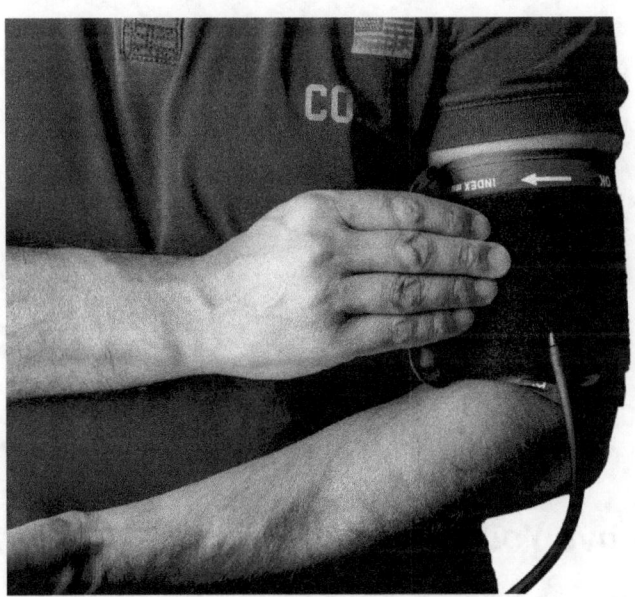

9. Carbohydrates Increase Energy Levels

Carbohydrates are the primary energy source of the body. Carbohydrates are eventually converted into glucose which is necessary for the production of ATP- the main energy currency of the body's cell. When you eat a diet low in carbohydrates, your body uses other alternative energy sources to produce glucose to provide you with energy. If you feel lethargic, a meal with high-quality carbohydrates is usually sufficient to get you out of the rut.

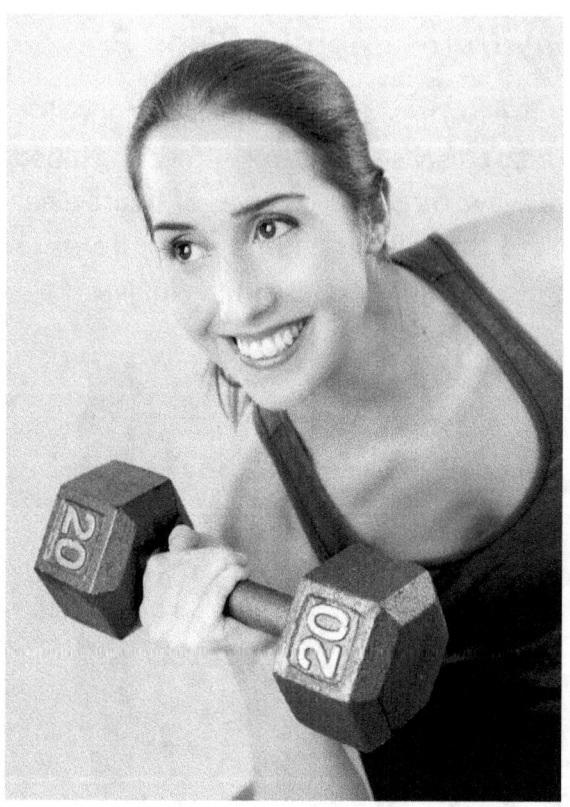

10. Can Improve Your Lifespan

Carbohydrate-rich foods stimulate two anabolic hormones, insulin and insulin-like growth factor 1 (IGF-1). IGF-1 plays an important role in cellular recovery and rejuvenation that helps keep your cellular age well beyond your chronological age. Moreover, carbohydrates stimulate growth hormone production, a key to slowing the aging process.

My Thoughts

Carbohydrates have many health benefits, but you need to make sure you are eating them in moderation. Although carbohydrates-containing food groups boast a host of vitamins and minerals required by the body, eating too much of any food group can result in weight gain. Consulting with your doctor can help you determine the amount of carbohydrates best for your health goals and existing health conditions.

CHAPTER 8

10 Healthy Carbohydrates You Must Eat for Health and Nutrition Benefits

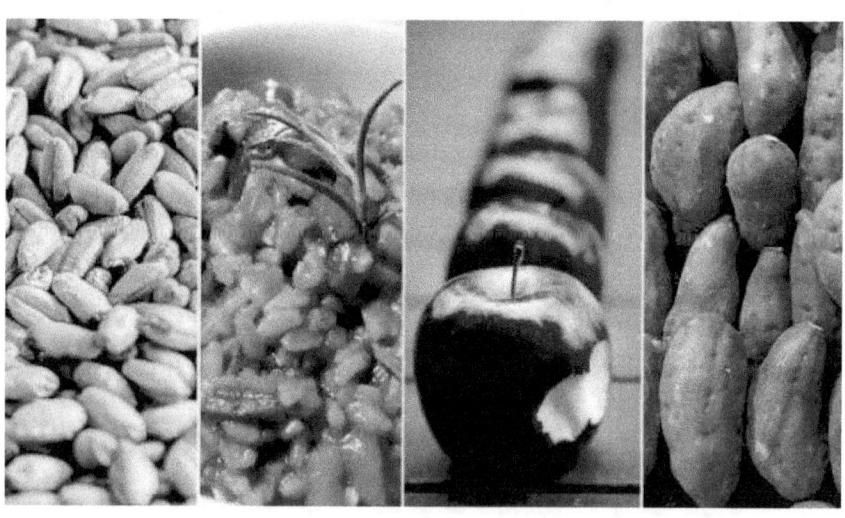

What are Carbs/Carbohydrates?

Carbohydrates are one of three macronutrients — along with proteins and fats — that your body requires daily.

Simple carbohydrates contain single monosaccharide units that are broken down quickly by the body to be used as energy. They are found in milk, milk products, fruit, and vegetables.

Complex carbohydrates are polysaccharides that are made up of complex chains of thousands of monosaccharide units. Complex carbohydrates digest slowly and take time to absorb into the body. They are found in whole grains, legumes, and starchy vegetables, like potatoes.

Why are Carbs Important?

The main function of carbohydrates is to supply energy to the body and brain. Carbohydrates improve brain power, reduce cancer risk, improve digestion and sleep pattern.

Below is the list of 10 high-quality carbohydrates that you must eat for health and nutrition benefits:

1. Whole Wheat

Unlike unhealthy refined wheat, which is processed to remove the bran and the germ, leaving only the endosperm, whole-wheat is made from the entire wheat kernels—bran, germ, and endosperm, which makes them highly nutritious.

Gluten is a group of proteins, occur with starch in the endosperm of wheat. As refined wheat or white flour only consist of endosperm, gluten is quite high in them. The amount of gluten present in 3 cups of whole wheat flour is equivalent to the amount of gluten present in 1 cup of white flour.

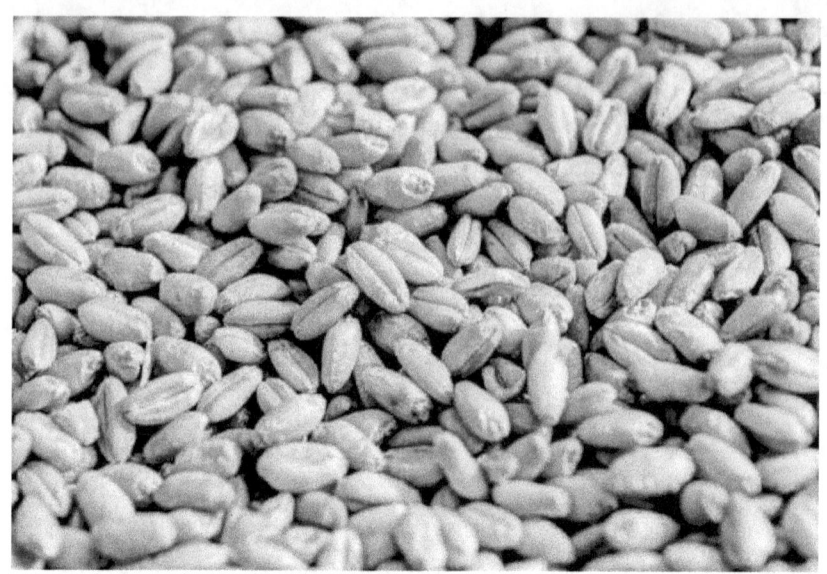

Whole wheat is a rich source of vitamin B6, dietary fiber, iron, calcium, potassium, magnesium, etc. Whole wheat has plenty of complex carbohydrates that give sustained energy. Bran from whole wheat provides dietary fiber, which reduces blood cholesterol levels and may lower the risk of heart disease.

100 g of whole wheat flour contains 72 g of total carbohydrates, of which 11 g is dietary fiber.

2. Brown Rice

Brown rice is whole-grain rice from which only inedible the husk (the outermost layer) is removed while from white rice, along with the hull, the bran layer, and the germ (the subsequent layers underneath the husk) are also removed, leaving only the starchy endosperm. During this removal and the further polishing process, several vitamins and minerals are lost.

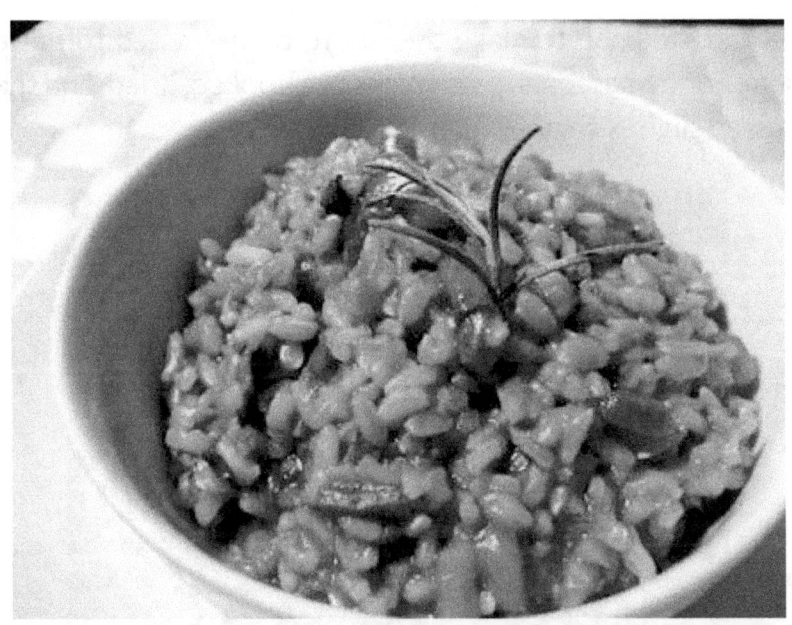

Brown rice is a good source of vitamin B1, B2, B6, magnesium, selenium, phosphorus, and high in fiber. Brown rice is considered a low glycemic index food as it digests more slowly, causing a lower change in blood sugar level. The soluble fiber in brown rice attaches to cholesterol particles and carries them out of the body, helping to reduce overall cholesterol and may help prevent the formation of blood clots.

100 g of raw brown rice contains 73 g of total carbohydrate, of which 3.52 g is dietary fiber.

3. Oats

Oat groats are the whole form of oats, mostly intact, hulled oat grains. Groats include the germ and fiber-rich bran portion of the grain, as well as the endosperm.

For steel-cut oats, whole oats groats are processed by chopping them into several pieces. For rolled oats, oats groats are first steamed to make them soft, then pressed to flatten them. For instant oats, oats groats pre-cooked, dried, and then pressed slightly thinner than rolled oats.

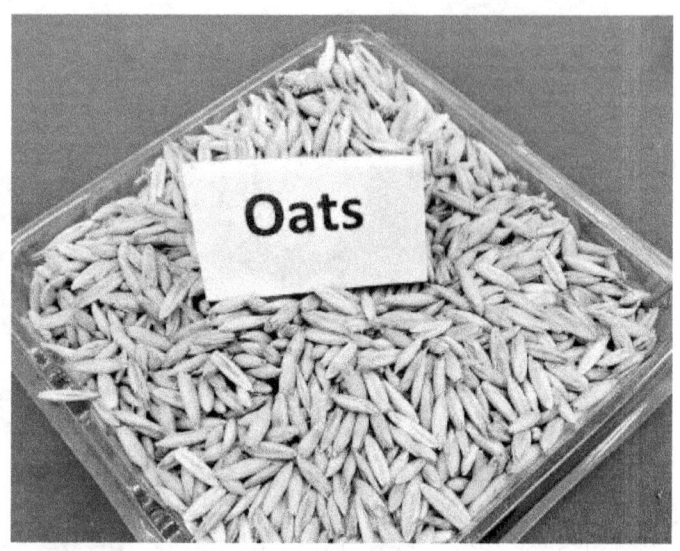

Steel-cut oats are marginally higher in fiber than rolled oats, while instant oats are the most highly processed variety and have relatively less nutritional value. Oat groats are the healthiest among all types of oats. You can coarsely grind oat groats into flour and use it to make bread, cookies, and chapati.

Oats are gluten-free whole grain and an excellent protein source, dietary fiber, antioxidants, vitamins, and minerals, especially manganese.

Oats are a rich source of water-soluble fiber β-glucan that helps keep cholesterol in check and managing diabetes. Oats promote healthy bacteria in the digestive tract, help fight cardiovascular disease and Type 2 diabetes.

100 grams of oats contain 66.3 grams of total carbohydrate, of which 11 grams is dietary fiber, 4 grams of soluble fiber β-

glucan.

4. Quinoa

Quinoa is a seed-producing flowering plant. It is pseudocereal which means unlike wheat and rice, quinoa is not grass but used in much the same way as cereals. Quinoa seed can be ground into flour and otherwise used as cereals.

Quinoa is high in complex carbohydrates, insoluble fiber, and protein which makes it very filling. It has complete protein, which means it contains all nine essential amino acids. It is also high in iron, magnesium, calcium, potassium, B vitamins, vitamin E, phosphorus, vitamin E, and antioxidants.

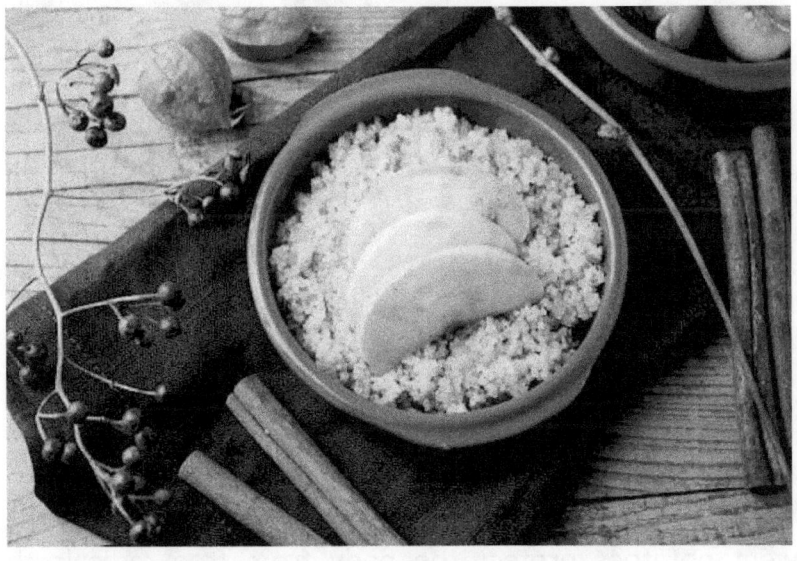

Another good part is that quinoa is gluten-free, so people with gluten intolerance can eat quinoa to meet their daily recommended carbs requirement.

Quinoa has anti-inflammatory properties. It regulates body temperature and aids enzyme activity.

100 g of raw quinoa contains 64.2 g of complex carbohydrates, of which 7 g is dietary fiber.

5. Sweet Potatoes

Sweet potatoes are rich in complex carbohydrates and are a great source of dietary fiber. They contain an array of vitamins such as vitamin C, vitamin B5, vitamin B6, and minerals, including iron, calcium, selenium, and manganese. One of the key health benefits of sweet potatoes is that they are high in beta-carotene, an antioxidant that converts into vitamin A in the body.

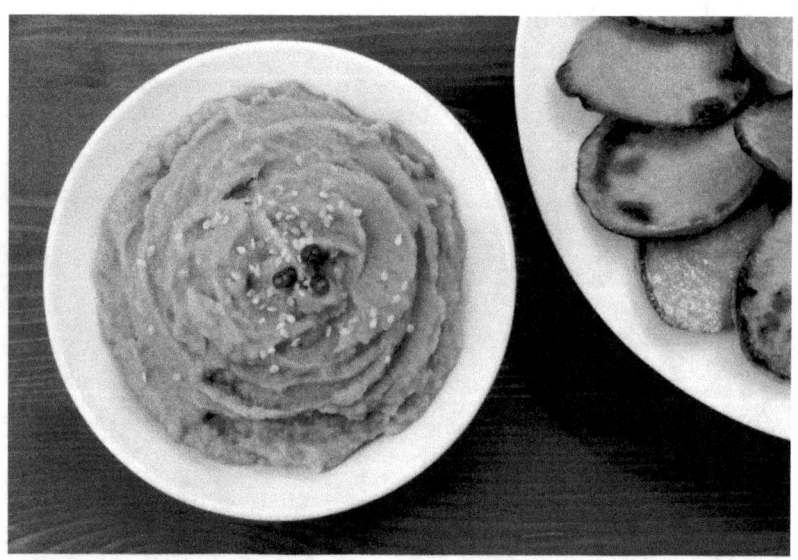

Sweet potatoes protect the body from free radicals that protect against cancer, support the immune system, and support healthy vision.

100 g of sweet potatoes contain 20 g of complex carbohydrates, of which 3 g is dietary fiber.

6. Boiled Potatoes

Boiled potatoes have a lower glycemic score than naked baked potatoes. Due to the low glycemic score, our body digests boiled potatoes more slowly, makes them easier to digest, and makes us feel full longer.

Boiled potatoes cooked with skin are very low in saturated fat, sodium and contain zero cholesterol.

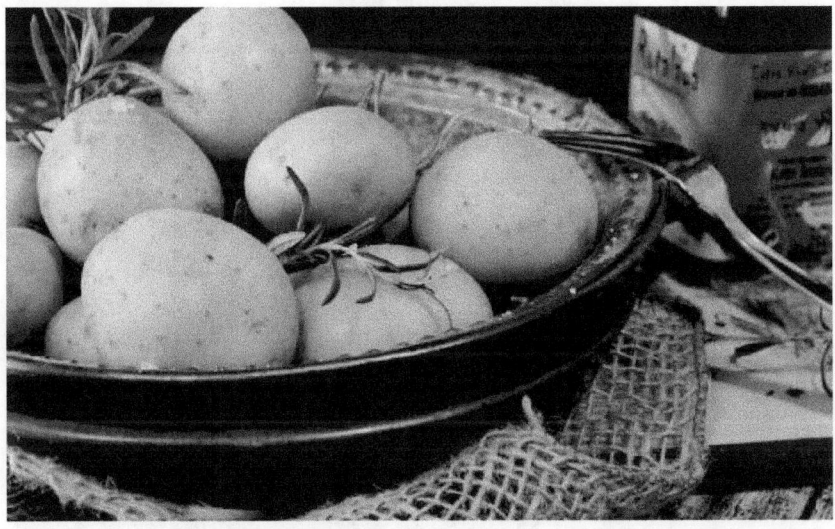

A large, boiled potato (with skin) is rich in vitamin B-complex. A boiled potato provides more than half of the recommended daily intake of vitamin B6. It is also a good source of vitamin C, copper, and potassium.

It contains resistant starch that improves gut health by making more good bacteria and less harmful bacteria in the gut. Moreover, boiled potatoes are gluten-free.

100 g of boiled potatoes contain 20 g of total carbohydrate, of which 1.6 g is dietary fiber.

7. Apples

For the maximum health benefits, eat the whole apple - both skin and flesh. Apples are extremely rich in dietary fiber. The soluble fiber content of apples may promote weight loss and gut health.

1 medium-sized apple contains 95 calories, and it takes 150 calories to digest an apple. It means you will burn an additional 50 calories simply by eating an apple.

Apples are highly rich in important antioxidants, flavonoids. The antioxidants and phytonutrients in apples help reduce the risk of developing diabetes, hypertension, heart disease, and cancer.

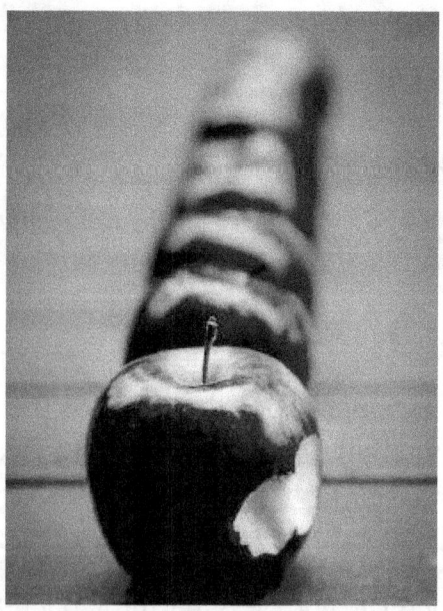

Other health benefits of apples include the prevention of stomach and liver disorders, anemia, gallstones, and constipation.

100 g of apples contain 14 g of total carbohydrate, of which 2.4 g is dietary fiber.

8. Bananas

Bananas are high in potassium, which promotes heart health. Eating these can help lower blood pressure and reduce the risk of cancer and asthma. Bananas are rich in fiber, calcium, vitamin B6, vitamin C, and various antioxidants and phytonutrients. Unripe bananas have a high content of resistant starch, which promotes intestinal health.

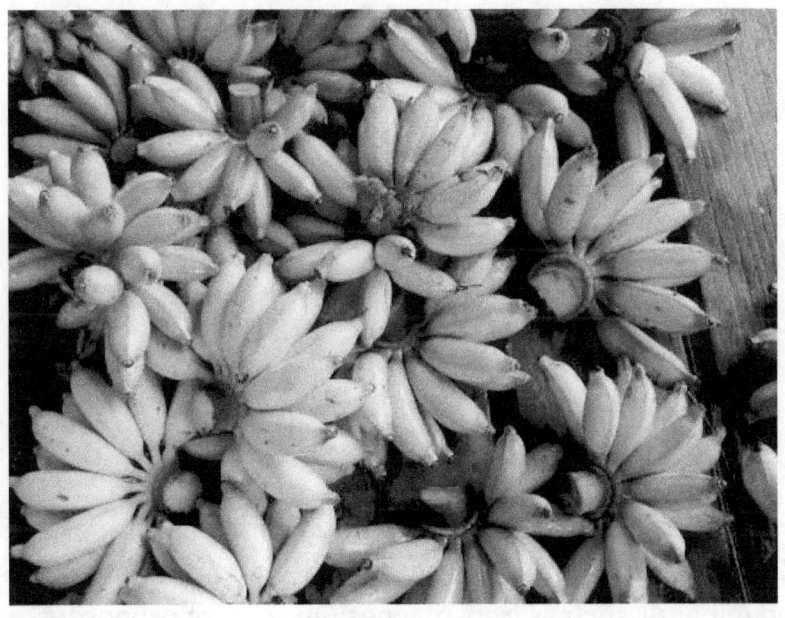

Bananas have a low glycemic index. Due to the high iron content, bananas are good for those suffering from anemia. Bananas have a decent amount of magnesium, which has been known to aid sound sleep.

100 g of bananas contain 23 g of total carbohydrate, of which 2.6 g is dietary fiber.

9. Chickpeas

Chickpeas are high in complex carbohydrates, making you feel full for a more extended period as they digest slowly. The starch found in chickpeas is digested slowly and supports more stabilized blood sugar levels. Chickpeas are high in protein which helps in weight loss. The fiber in chickpeas absorb water and attach to toxins and waste as they move through the digestive system, forming stool containing toxins and waste that must be removed from the body.

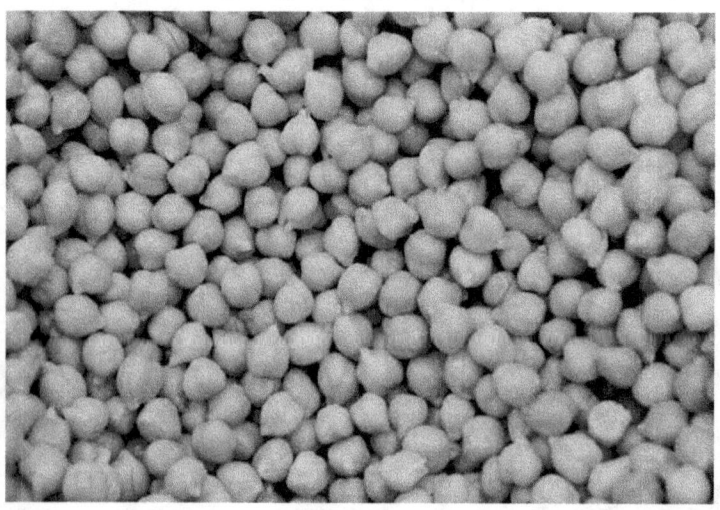

They are a rich source of the essential vitamin B complex (B1, B2, B3, B6, B12), vitamin A, vitamin C, vitamin K, antioxidants, and minerals such as iron, magnesium, zinc, phosphorous, and folate.

100 g of chickpeas contain 61 g of total carbohydrate, of which 17 g is dietary fiber.

Read 10 Nutrient Combinations You Should Eat for Maximum Health Benefits in the book Eat to Prevent and Control Disease.

10. Kidney Beans

Kidney beans contain both soluble and insoluble fiber that keeps your digestive system running smoothly. Soluble fiber can bind cholesterol in the intestine and remove it from the body, and insoluble fiber prevents constipation by adding bulk to the stool.

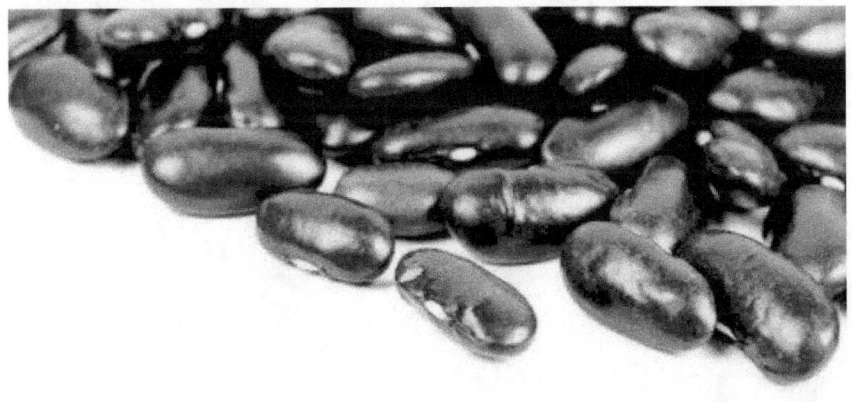

They contain slow carbohydrates, which means the carbohydrates break down and are absorbed from the intestines, slowly avoiding sudden blood sugar spikes. Antioxidants found in kidney beans help combat cancer. Additionally, calcium and magnesium in kidney beans can prevent osteoporosis and strengthen the bones. Kidney beans are the richest plant-based protein source that boosts muscle mass.

100 g of kidney beans contain 6 g of total carbohydrate, of which 25 g is dietary fiber.

Conclusion

The health benefits of high-quality carbohydrate-rich foods are countless. Do not confuse healthy carbs with refined, processed carbs like cookies and donuts. One should not depend on refined carbohydrates to meet the recommended daily intake of carbohydrates. Include high-quality carbohydrates in your diet for a healthy life. Carbohydrate-restricted diets carry potential risks of osteoporosis and cancer incidence. But keep in mind that eating carbs in excess can lead to weight gain.

Preventive Measures

Vegetarian diets can prevent you from many diseases. It adds valuable and healthy years to your life. However, some essential nutrients are found in lesser quantity in plant-based vegetarian foods, having said that there is no essential nutrient which can't be found in vegetarian foods. In general, vegetarians' diet consists of 60–70% of carbohydrates, and the protein intake of vegetarians is less than that of non-vegetarians, which sometimes causes protein deficiency. Therefore, as a vegetarian, you must eat an adequate amount of protein in your diet daily. You can find the **list of protein-rich foods** in chapter 4 of this book.

Other health issues that vegetarians face are:

Iron Deficiency Anemia

Vitamin B12 Deficiency

Fortunately, prevention from these conditions doesn't cost you physician fees. In fact, prevention from these conditions doesn't even require fancy costly foods, and you can prevent them by smart eating. All you need to add some simple foods to your diet, and you are fit inside out. Let's discuss both conditions one by one in detail.

CHAPTER 9

10 Power Foods to Get Rid of Anemia

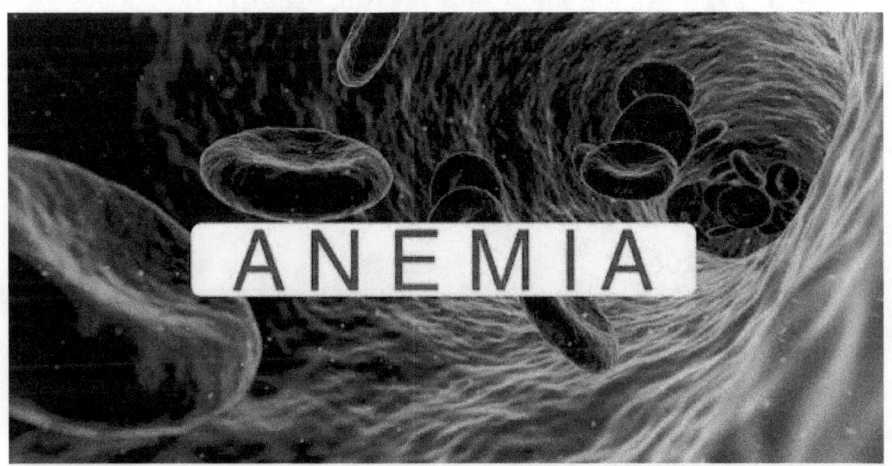

What is Anemia?

Iron Deficiency Anemia is a common condition in which there is a deficiency of red blood cells or hemoglobin in the blood.

Iron deficiency anemia is caused due to insufficient iron in the body. Without enough iron, the body can't produce enough hemoglobin in red blood cells. Hemoglobin is the main part of red blood cells and binds oxygen. Hemoglobin in the blood carries oxygen from the lungs or gills to the rest of the body.

Cause of Anemia

Iron deficiency is amongst the most common nutritional deficiencies and the most common cause of anemia. However, other conditions, such as vitamin B12, folate, and vitamin A deficiencies, can also cause anemia.

Inadequate iron intake due to poor diet, blood loss through heavy periods, inflammatory bowel disease, and increased blood requirement during pregnancy lead to anemia.

Symptoms of Anemia

Iron deficiency anemia symptoms may include:

- Fatigue
- Dizziness
- Cold hands and feet
- Weakness
- Pale skin
- Irregular heartbeats
- Shortness of breath, particularly with exercise

With the proper diet rich in iron, one can get rid of anemia.

Heme Iron and Non-Heme Iron

The two forms of dietary iron are

Heme Iron

Non-Heme Iron

Iron from animal proteins like seafood, meat, poultry, and fish are known as Heme iron.

The iron that comes from plants is known as non-heme iron and is found in plant-based foods like grains, fruits, beans, vegetables, nuts, seeds, and iron-fortified foods such as oats.

Vitamin C helps your stomach absorb iron, and you get maximum health benefits. Try to eat non-heme iron foods combined with vitamin C (for example, a glass of lemon juice, orange, berries, kiwi fruit, tomatoes, and capsicum) to increase absorption of iron.

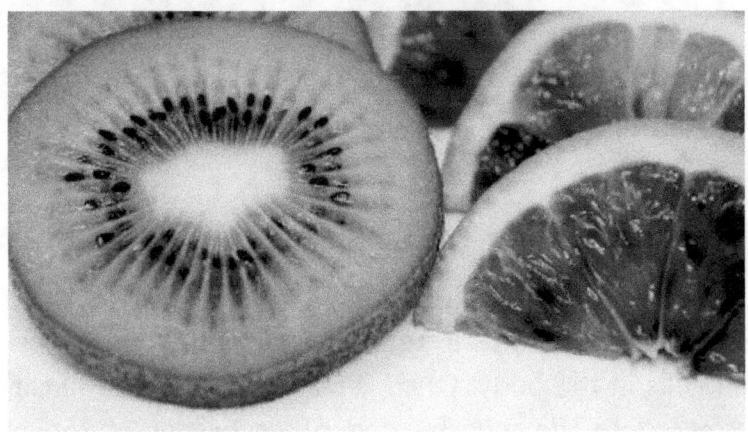

As this is a vegetarian zone, we will discuss vegetarian options in detail.

Below is the list of 10 power foods to get rid of anemia:

1. Spinach

Spinach is rich in iron, beta-carotene, calcium, vitamin B9 and C, and fiber. Regular consumption of spinach can prevent anemia. Spinach is much better than red meat as it provides fewer calories and is fat and cholesterol-free. To get maximum health benefits, include spinach in your daily diet. Make sure to combine vitamin-C-rich foods such as citrus fruits with spinach to improve absorption.

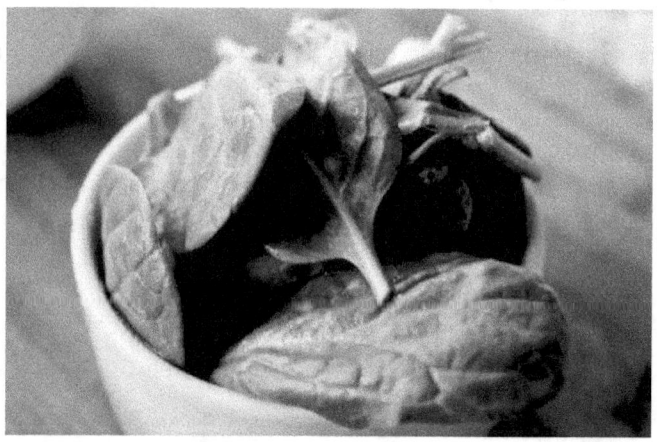

2. Beetroot

Beetroot is loaded with iron and vitamin C, which is good for anemia. Beetroot helps in repairing and reactivating the red blood cells in the body. Once repaired, oxygen can easily be transferred to the muscles and other tissues of the body. Adding beetroot in any form to your everyday diet will help to fight anemia easily.

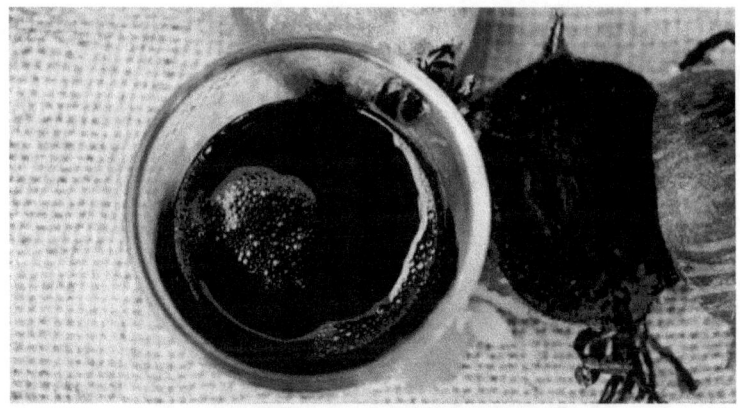

3. Lentils

Legumes—especially lentils—are great for anemia, as just a half-cup has around 20% of iron that your body needs for the day. Legumes are also high in folate, potassium, magnesium, and fiber that fill you up and help lower cholesterol levels, stabilize your blood sugar, and even aid weight loss.

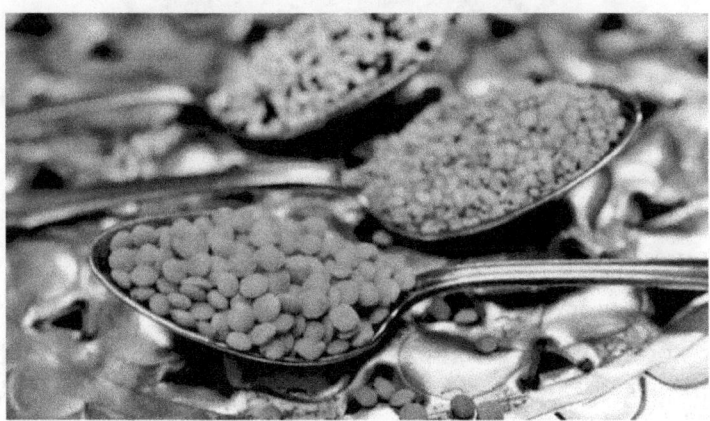

4. Honey

Honey is among the most widely used sweetener with enormous health benefits. Honey is a rich source of iron. Along with iron, the presence of copper and magnesium in honey increases the concentration of hemoglobin in your blood, thereby treating anemia. Mixing one tablespoon of honey and some lemon juice in a glass of lukewarm water, drinking on an empty stomach daily in the morning helps in fighting anemia.

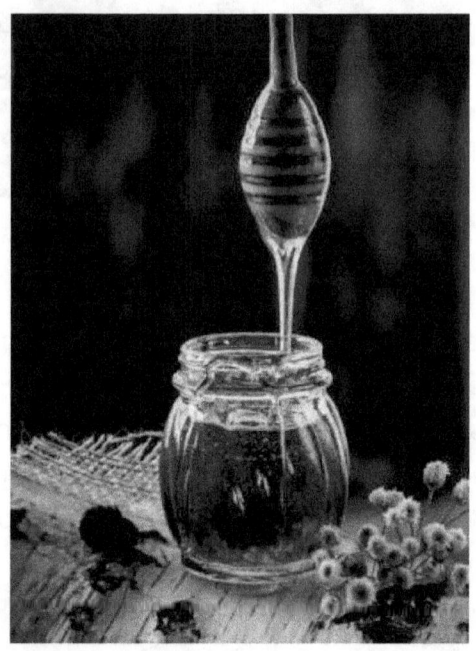

5. Jaggery/ Panela

Jaggery is commonly known as gur in India and panela in the rest of the world. Regular intake of jaggery helps combat anemia. Jaggery is unrefined sugar. It is the purest form of sugar and is prepared in iron vessels with fruit juices without any addition of synthetic chemicals. It is rich in iron and folate that helps prevent anemia. Taking jaggery with ginger juice helps in better absorption of iron.

6. Chickpeas

Chickpeas are high in protein and fiber. Chickpeas are the iron powerhouse for vegetarians and contain several vital vitamins and minerals.

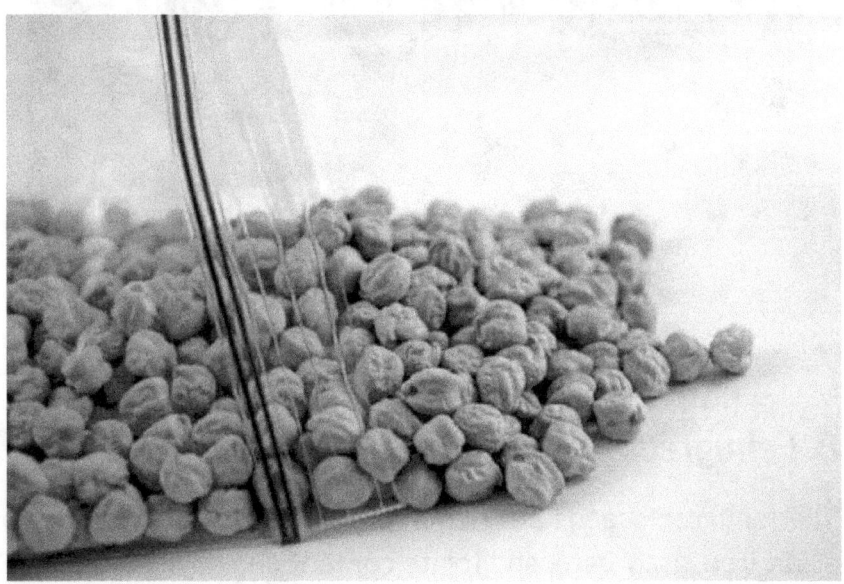

They are rich in iron, folate, and vitamin C, which are necessary to synthesize hemoglobin. The higher protein and iron content of chickpeas make them a smart option for vegetarians. Add lemon juice to hummus for better iron absorption.

*Read 10 Superfoods you should eat every day in the book Eat to Prevent and Control Disease.

7. Pumpkin Seeds

Pumpkin seeds are rich in iron, antioxidants, zinc, magnesium, and many other nutrients. Only a handful of pumpkin seeds every two days can help strengthen the immune system and prevent anemia. Add the roasted pumpkin seeds to morning cereal, bread, yogurt, or salad topping.

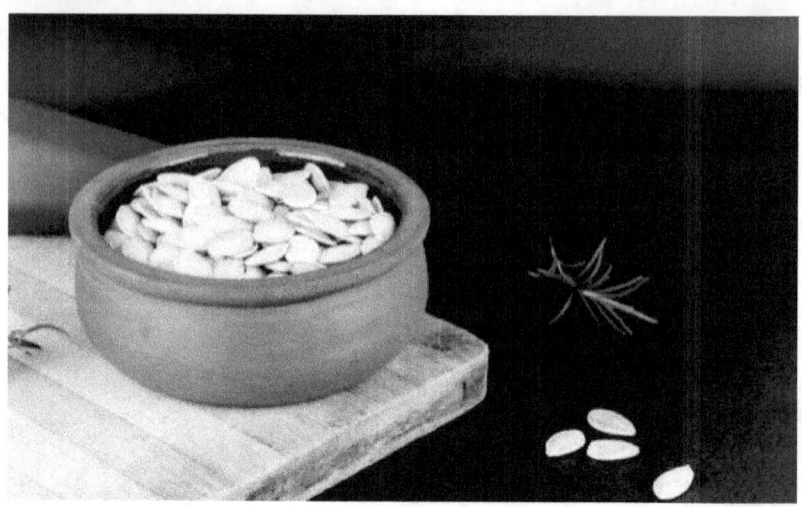

8. Fenugreek

The fenugreek seeds are rich in protein with essential amino acids, iron, ascorbate, and folate content and have restorative and nutritive properties. Fenugreek helps prevent and cure anemia and maintain good health for long periods. Fenugreek leaves help in blood formation. Fenugreek seeds are a valuable cure for anemia, being rich in iron.

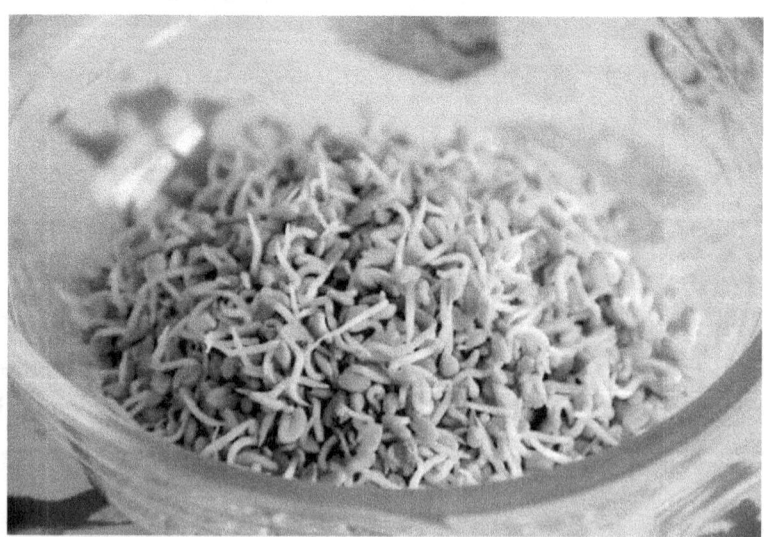

9. Soybeans

Soybeans are a great source of iron. Soybeans are high in protein and fiber and low in fat that fights anemia. They're an excellent source of important minerals like copper, which helps keep your blood vessels and immune system healthy. It is also high in manganese, an essential nutrient involved in many chemical processes in the body.

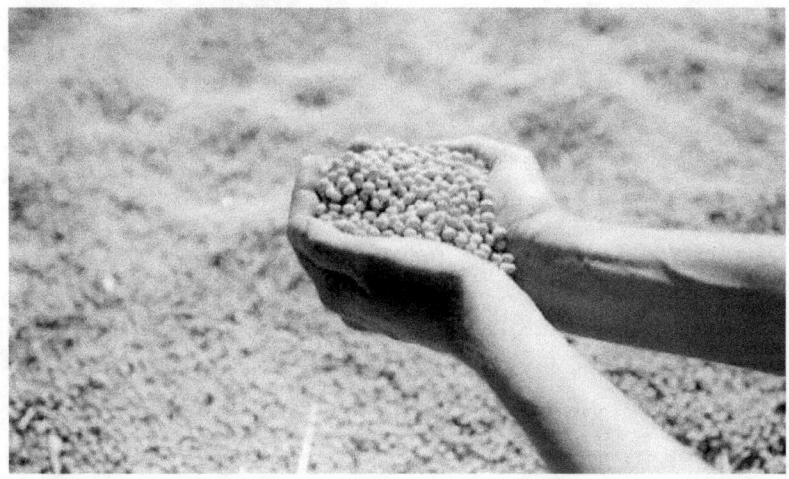

10. Sesame Seeds

The iron in sesame seeds can keep the immune system functioning properly and prevent iron-deficient anemia. Especially the black sesame seeds are a great source of iron. The seeds are packed with essential nutrients, like copper, phosphorus, vitamin E, and zinc as well. One quarter cup size serving of sesame seeds can provide 30% of the daily iron requirement.

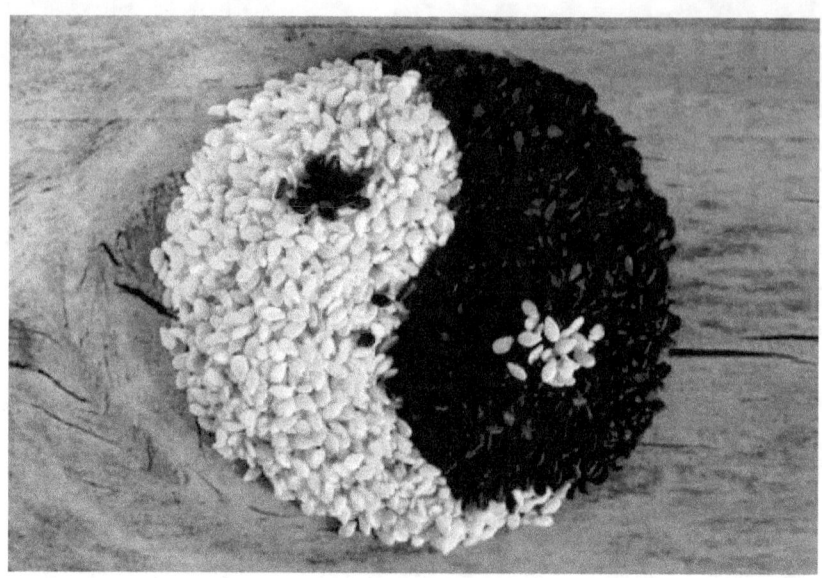

Conclusion

Body cannot produce iron on its own, which is an important mineral. It plays a crucial role in cell growth and differentiation. Therefore, consuming an iron-rich diet regularly is essential. Remember to include a vitamin C source when eating non-heme plant sources of iron to boost its absorption in the body. Girls should increase iron consumption during periods to combat blood loss. Similarly, women who are pregnant should increase their iron consumption. They are at a higher risk of developing anemia because the body produces an excess of blood to provide nutrients to the baby.

CHAPTER 10

Top 10 Foods for Vegetarians to Prevent Vitamin B12 Deficiency

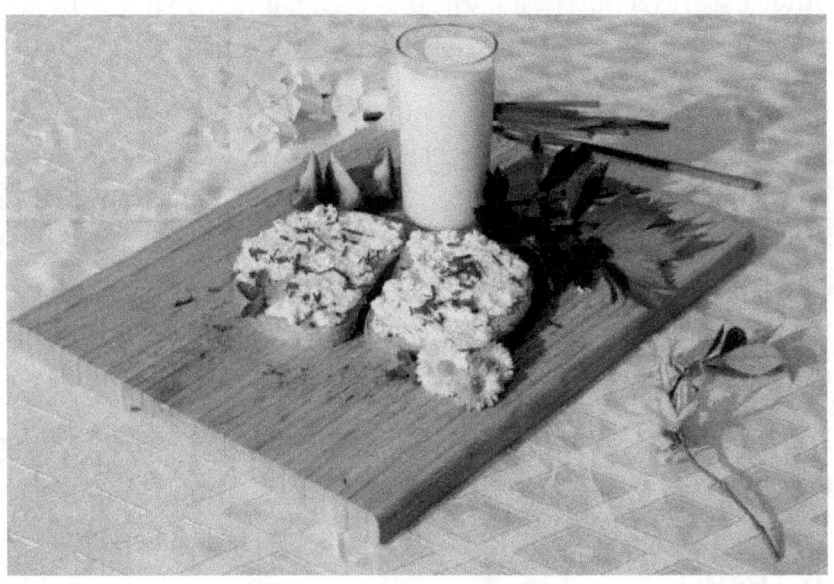

If you feel fatigued, depressed, and irritated all the time. If you hear a ringing sound in 1 or both ears or experiencing memory trouble and poor balance, you may have Vitamin B12

Deficiency, also known as Cobalamin Deficiency. Protein foods are the primary sources of vitamin B12, including animal meats and fish, which is why vegetarians often lack vitamin B12.

What is Vitamin B12 and Why is it Important?

Vitamin B12 or cobalamin is a water-soluble vitamin. It is an essential nutrient important in the nervous system's normal functioning, helps make DNA, the genetic material in human cells, and keeps blood cells healthy. Vitamin B12 deficiency may lead to a reduction in healthy red blood cells that may result in anemia. The Dietary Reference Intake (DRI), for adult men and women, is 2.4 micrograms of vitamin B12 in a day. Like other essential nutrients, Vitamin B12 cannot be made by the body. Instead, it should be obtained from food.

If your vitamin B12 level is quite low, you have to take supplements or vitamin B12 injections, whichever your physician advises. But if you have borderline vitamin B12 deficiency or want to prevent it in the future, you must start eating vitamin B12 rich foods. Although vitamin B12 is mainly found in animal sources, there are some vegetarian options to prevent its deficiency.

I am listing below the top 10 vitamin B12 rich foods for vegetarians.

1. Yogurt

Eating yogurt daily is an excellent way to get more vitamin B12. Yogurt has the highest absorption of vitamin B12, between 50% and 75%. Yogurt is also a good source of folate and vitamin B6. Go for low-fat, unsweetened plain yogurt to avoid weight gain.

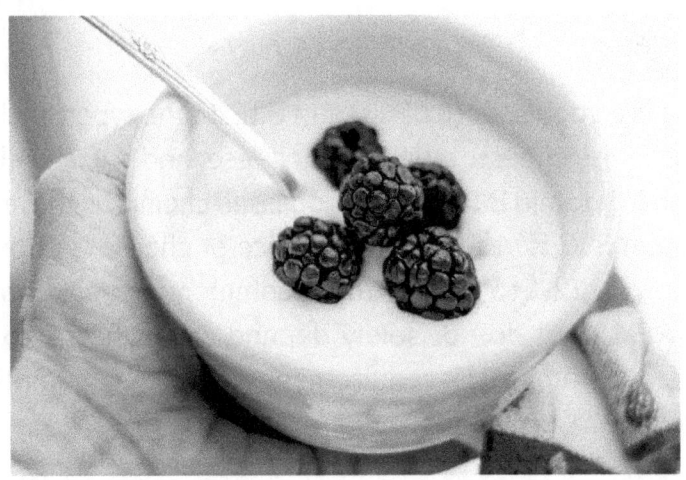

2. Cow's Milk

Milk is another excellent source of vitamin B12, and adequate consumption may help prevent vitamin B12 deficiency. About 2 cups of 250 ml of milk per day can get you the recommended daily intake of vitamin B12. It is loaded with other nutrients such as calcium, protein, potassium, and phosphorus. Have it with breakfast cereal, and you will get more Vitamin B12.

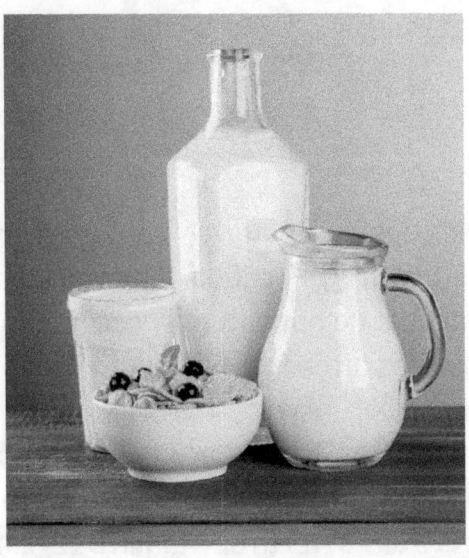

3. Cheese

Cheese is a good source of vitamin B12. Some types of cheese, such as Swiss cheese, mozzarella cheese, and cottage cheese, are high in vitamin B12. Avoid processed cheese as the amount of vitamin B12 is very low in it. 1 slice of cheese is enough to provide you 22% to 36% of the recommended daily intake of vitamin B12 but do not solely depend upon cheese to fulfill your daily vitamin B12 requirement as large consumption of cheese may make you fat.

4. Soy Milk

As such, soy milk does not naturally contain vitamin B12, but it can be fortified with it. Fortified food means that food has added nutrients that do not naturally occur in that food. In the case of soy milk, it is often fortified with vitamin B12 - be sure to check the label. Avoid flavored ones and choose unsweetened varieties as they are more natural and free of void calories, that is, sugar. With just one cup of fortified soy milk, you can get a day's worth of vitamin B12 (2.4 micrograms).

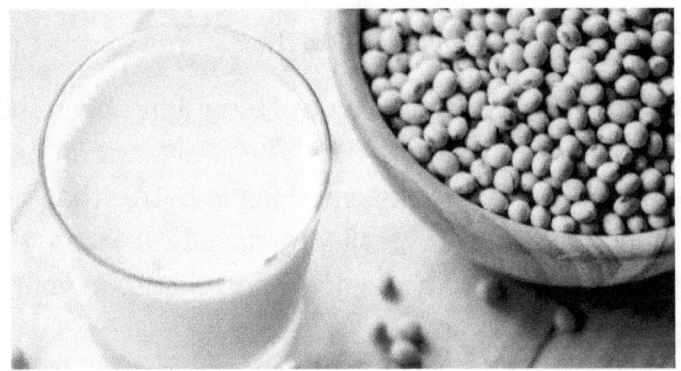

5. Tempeh

Tempeh is made by a culturing and controlled fermentation process that binds soybeans into a cake form. Bacterial contamination during tempeh production may contribute to the increased vitamin B12 content of tempeh. The amount of vitamin B12 present in tempeh is relatively low in comparison to milk products. Therefore, you shouldn't solely rely on it to meet your daily recommended vitamin B12 requirement. Still, it can boost your plant-based protein intake, giving you plenty of fiber with no cholesterol or saturated fat.

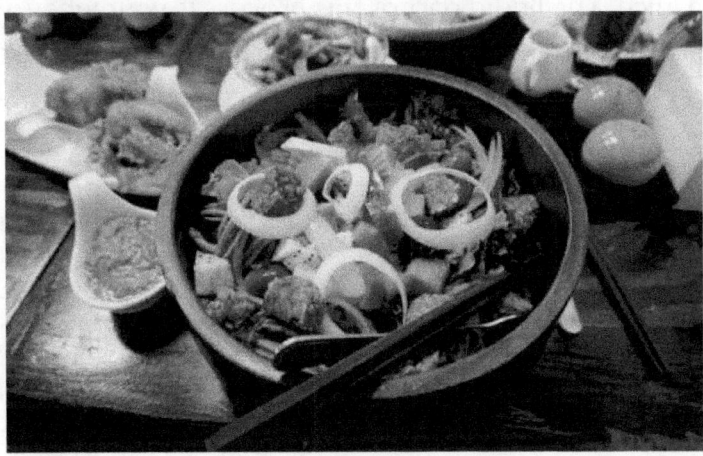

6. Dried Shiitake Mushroom

Dried Shiitake Mushrooms, a type of fungi, have been shown to contain significant levels of B12. These are not an excellent source of vitamin B12, but something is better than nothing. You can increase your overall vitamin B12 intake by adding dried shiitake mushrooms, tempeh, and cheese in your wraps and stuffing.

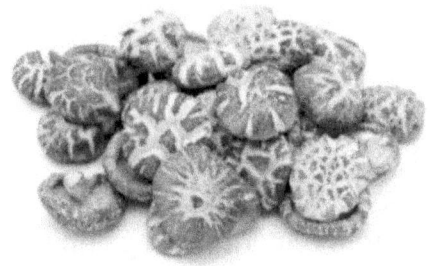

7. Whey Protein

Whey protein is a great source of vitamin B12. You can make your own whey protein at home by curdling boiled milk with lemon juice. The liquid part of this process is your whey, which is rich in vitamin B12 and a great source of protein for vegetarians. Use this whey in your pancake batter or add it to your pasta recipes to get the full health benefits of whey.

8. Cereal

Breakfast cereal such as muesli and granola is a good source of vitamin B12. If you don't enjoy your cereal with milk, eat cereal as a snack during office break time or try it as a late-night snack. Be sure to go for unsweetened varieties to avoid unnecessary fat in your diet.

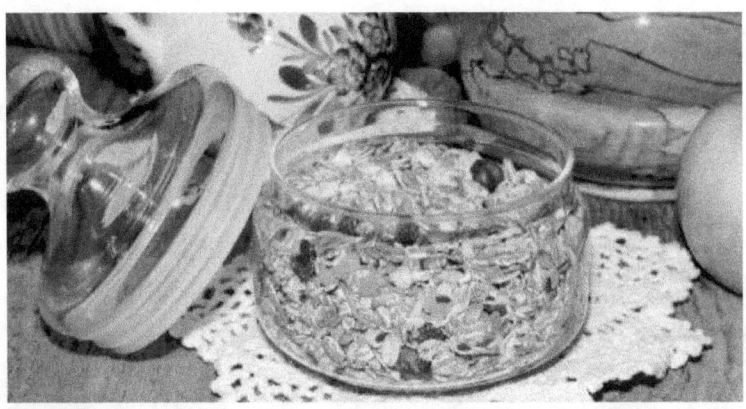

9. Vanilla Ice Cream

Ice cream is made of milk, and vitamin B12 is naturally found in milk, making ice cream a good source of vitamin B12. Not only this, but ice cream also contains vitamin A, B complex, C, D, K, and E, calcium, and protein. On the other hand, it is high in cholesterol and saturated fat. Therefore, it should be consumed in a lesser amount for overall health. A single cup serving of vanilla ice cream contains 20 percent of the recommended daily intake of vitamin B12.

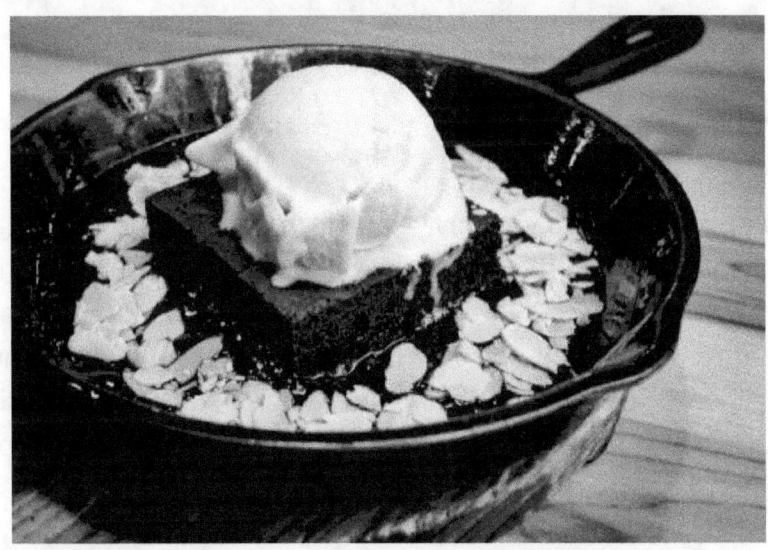

10. Rice Milk

Rice milk is a good source of vitamin B12. It has zero saturated fat and rich in vitamin A, D, calcium, magnesium, potassium, and iron. You can make it at your home by finely blending a ½ cup of cooked brown rice with 2 cups of water. For extra smooth rice milk, simply pass the liquid through the strainer to remove any lumps. It tastes best when served chilled.

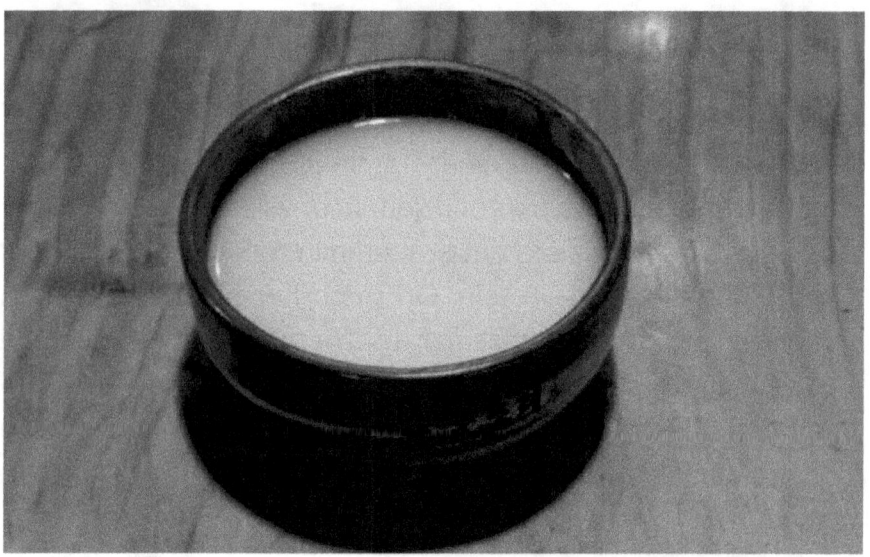

Conclusion

Vitamin B12 deficiency is not very uncommon among vegetarians, but all you have to do is make some little changes to your diet or, more accurately, include more vitamin B12 rich foods in your diet. With a few simple changes, you can have great results. It will not only prevent vitamin B12 deficiency, but it will also prevent anemia. Since vitamin B12 foods are rich in protein, you will get the double benefit of a healthy nervous system, healthy skin, and many more.

CHAPTER 11

Recipes

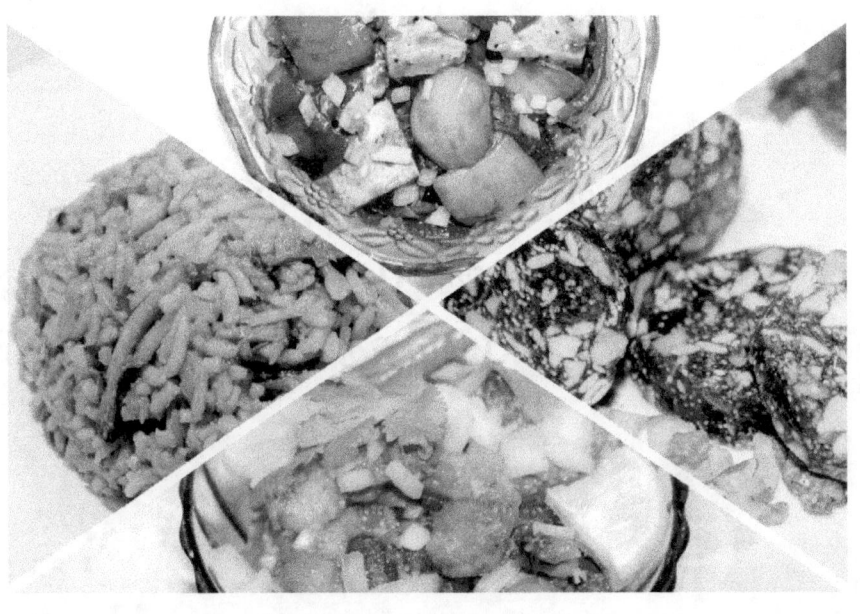

Chilli Tofu

Beans in Schezwan Sauce

Mushroom Fried Pulao

Khajur Roll

Chilli Tofu

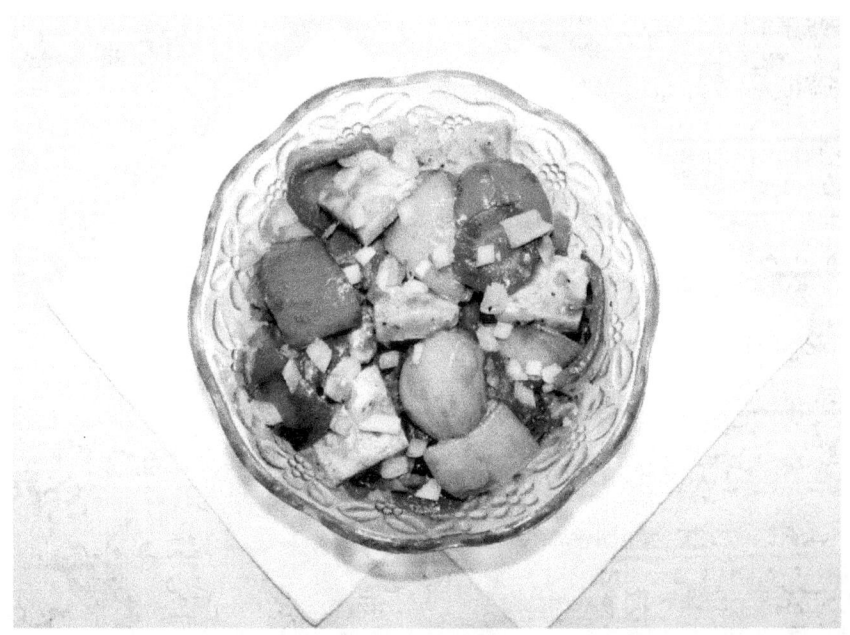

Serves 2

Ingredients

Tofu: 100 gm

Capsicum: 100 gm

Carrot: 100 gm

Onion: 100 gm

Chopped garlic: 2 tablespoons

Chopped ginger: 1 teaspoon

Red chili sauce: 1 tablespoon

Soy sauce: 1 tablespoon

Tomato sauce: 1 tablespoon

White Sesame seeds: 1 teaspoon

Black pepper powder: ½ teaspoon

Dry mango powder: 1 teaspoon (optional)

Vinegar: 1 teaspoon

Corn flour: 1 tablespoon

Salt to Taste

Water: 50 ml + 2 tablespoons (if required)

Mustard oil: 2 tablespoons

Spring onion: To garnish

Method

1. Cut tofu into 1-inch cubes and sprinkle some salt and pepper over it.

2. Chop capsicum, carrot, and onion in 1-inch cubes.

3. Mix 1 tablespoon of cornflour in 50 ml of water and keep aside.

4. In a bowl, mix soy sauce, red chili sauce, and tomato sauce. Keep aside.

5. Heat mustard oil in a pan. Add sesame seeds. Once splutter, add chopped ginger and garlic.

6. Now turn the flame to high. Cook for 1-2 min. Keep the flame

on high for the rest of the steps.

7. Add capsicum and cook for 2 to 3 min and then add carrot and cook for 2-3 min. Gradually mix so that veggies cook evenly. Don't overcook. Veggies should be crisp and crunchy, not soggy.

8. Add onion. Cook on high flame for 3-4 min or till it becomes slightly translucent. Do not overcook otherwise it will become soggy.

9. Turn the flame to low and add sauce mix. Add black pepper, salt, and ½ teaspoon dry mango powder or vinegar. Mix well.

10. Add the cornflour paste and turn the flame to high. Once it starts boiling and the sauce become thick, add tofu pieces. Mix well. Cook for another 2 -3 min till tofu absorbs all the flavors.

11. Turn off the flame. Take it into a bowl and sprinkle some dry mango powder. Garnish with spring onion and enjoy it while it still hot.

Note: As MSG (Monosodium glutamate) is not a healthy option, it is not added to this recipe. You can replace mustard oil with any other oil if it is not available to you. Adding dry mango powder is optional. We are using mustard oil and dry mango powder combination to have a similar taste as MSG.

Beans in Schezwan Sauce

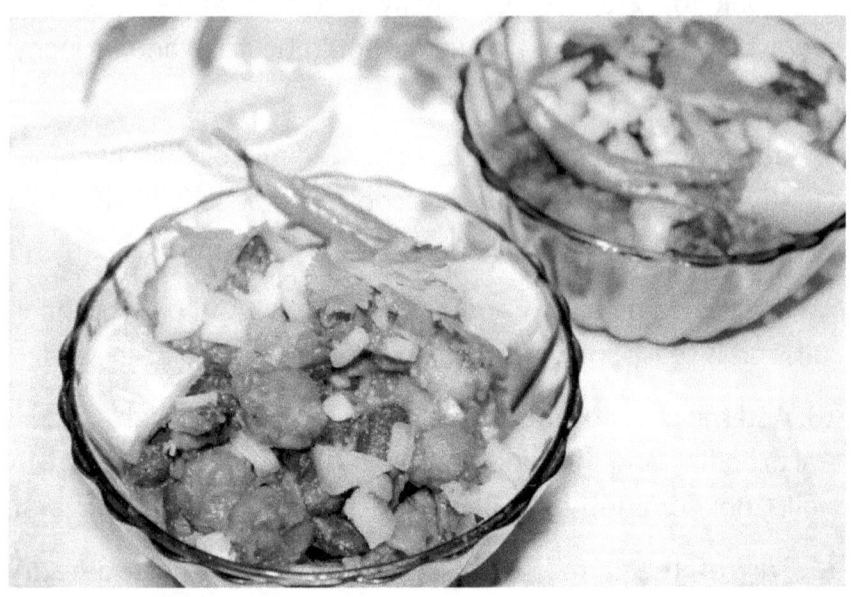

Serves 2

Ingredients:

Boiled chickpeas: 1½ cup

Boiled kidney beans: ½ cup

Boiled potatoes: 1 medium

Onion: 1 medium

Cumin: 1 teaspoon

Salt to Taste

Chopped garlic: 2 tablespoons

Chopped ginger: 1 tablespoon

Schezwan sauce: 2 tablespoons

Coriander leaves: To garnish

Green chilies: To garnish

Lemon: To garnish

Chopped onion: To garnish

Oil: 1 tablespoon

Method:

1. Heat oil in a pan. Add cumin. Sauté for 2 mins.

2. Add garlic and ginger. Cook for 2 mins on high flame.

3. Add chopped onion and cook till it becomes translucent.

4. Add chickpeas and kidney beans. Cook for 2 mins.

5. Add schezwan sauce and salt. Mix well.

6. Add chopped boiled potatoes. Cook on high for 2 mins.

7. Add 2 tablespoons of water if it looks dry. Cook for 5 mins on low to medium flame.

8. Turn off the flame. Garnish with chopped onion, coriander leaves, green chilies, and lemon. Enjoy beans in schezwan sauce with evening tea.

Mushroom Fried Pulao

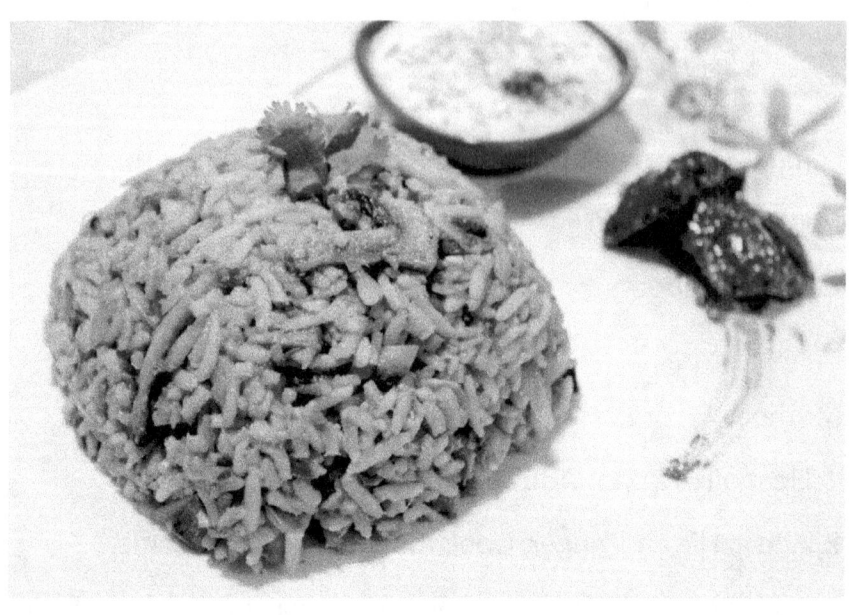

Serves: 2

Ingredients:

Mushroom: 100 gm

Cooked brown rice: 2 cups

Cumin: 1 tablespoon

Asafoetida: a pinch

Cashew nuts: 5 broken

Raisins: 8-10

Onion: 2 medium size

Chopped Garlic: 2 tablespoons

Tomatoes: 2 medium size

Yogurt: 2 tablespoons

Salt to Taste

Turmeric powder: 1 teaspoon

Coriander-cumin powder: 1 teaspoon

Garam masala: 1 teaspoon

Oil: 2 tablespoons

Method:

1. Warm oil in a pan. Add cashew nuts and fry till golden brown. Remove cashew nuts from oil.

2. Add asafetida and cumin to the remaining oil. Cook for a min.

3. Add garlic and cook for a min. Don't burn the garlic. Add onion and cook for about 5 mins on low to medium flame or till it becomes translucent.

4. Add tomatoes and salt. Salt will soften the tomatoes faster. Cover with a lid and cook for about 10-15 mins at low flame. Tomatoes should be softened completely. Mash the tomatoes with a spatula.

5. Add turmeric, coriander-cumin powder, red chili powder, and garam masala. Mix well. If it looks dry, add 2-3 tablespoons of water. Cover with lid and cook for 5 mins or till it leaves oil. Few drops of oil will be visible on the sides of the tomato mix.

6. Add chopped mushrooms. Mix well and cover it with a lid. Let

the mushrooms absorb all the spices.

7. Turn the flame to low and add yogurt. Mix for 2 mins. Add cooked brown rice and mix gently. Cook on medium-high flame for 5 mins.

8. Add cashew nuts and raisins. Mix well.

9. Turn off the flame, sprinkle coriander leaves and cover with a lid and leave for 10 mins.

10. Now it is ready to serve. Enjoy mushroom fried pulao with curd and pickle.

Note: Whenever using brown rice, always leave the dish covered for at least 10 mins. Brown rice absorbs flavors slowly as compared to white rice. Covering ensure the flavor to lock in the brown rice.

Khajur Roll

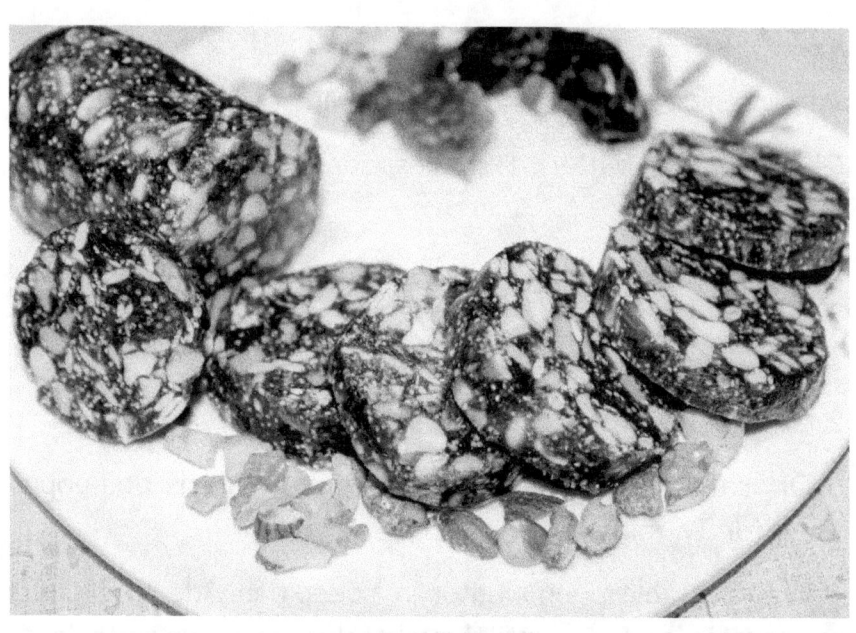

For 20 rolls

Ingredients:

Dates (deseeded): 1½ cup

Dried figs: ½ cup

Almonds: ¼ cup

Cashews: ¼ cup

Walnuts: ¼ cup

Pistachio: ¼ cup

White sesame: 1 tablespoon

Melon seeds: 1 tablespoon

Pumpkin seeds: 1 tablespoon

Poppy seeds: 1 teaspoon

Ghee (Clarified butter): 1½ tablespoons

Method:

1. Chop almonds, cashews, walnuts, and pistachio finely.

2. Grind dates and fig without using any water.

3. Dry roast sesame, melon seeds, pumpkin seeds, and poppy seeds for 3-5 mins.

4. Warm ½ tablespoon of ghee in a deep pan. Add all the nuts and roast in low flame until they slightly turn brown and release an aromatic smell.

5. Remove the nuts from heat. Add 1 tablespoon of ghee to the same pan.

6. Add dates and fig mixture. Mix well. Cover with a lid and let it soften for about 2 minutes.

7. Remove the lid and cook for about 5-7 min. Add nuts and seeds to it. Mix well and bind the mixture together by pressing it with a spatula.

8. Turn off the flame. Let it cool for 2 min. Take out the mixture on a plate. Grease your palm with ghee so that the mix doesn't stick to your palm. Now give the mixture a cylinder shape. Wrap it in with a cling film. Refrigerate the roll for 1 hour.

9. Take out the roll from the fridge. Remove the cling film. Grease a knife and cut the roll into small pieces.

10. Store in a clean and dry place for up to 2 weeks.

About the Author

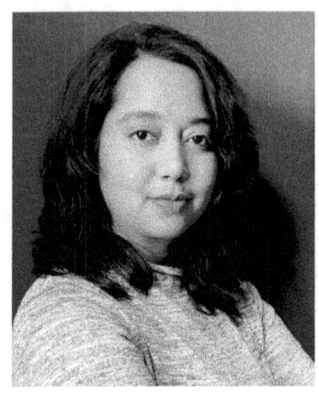

La Fonceur is the author of the book series *Eat So What!*, *Secret of Healthy Hair*, and *Eat to Prevent and Control Disease*. She is a health blogger and a dance artist. She has a master's degree in Pharmacy. She specialized in Pharmaceutical Technology and worked as a research scientist in the research and development department. She has published an article titled "Techniques for Producing Biotechnology-Derived Products of Pharmaceutical Use" in the Pharmtechmedica Journal. She is also a registered pharmacist. Being a research scientist, she has worked closely with drugs. Based on her experience, she believes that one can prevent most diseases with nutritious vegetarian foods and a healthy lifestyle.

Note from La Fonceur

Dear Reader,

Thank you for reading *Eat So What! The Power of Vegetarianism*. I hope you have found this book helpful.

If you liked the book, please leave a short review online telling why you enjoyed reading it. This will help other health-conscious readers find this book. Your help in spreading awareness is gratefully received.

Join my mailing list at www.eatsowhat.com/esw-newsletter to receive updates on my new release.

Also, read how foods that work with the same mechanism as medicines can naturally prevent and control disease in *Eat to Prevent and Control Disease*.

If you are looking for a permanent solution to your hair problems, read *Secret of Healthy Hair*.

This book is the extension of my previously released Nutrition Guide *Eat So What! Smart Ways to Stay Healthy*, which tells how the vegetarian diet is the solution to most general health problems, including skin, digestion, and weight gain issues.

All of my books are available in eBook, paperback, and hardcover editions. Happy reading!

Regards

La Fonceur

All Books by La Fonceur

Full-length books:

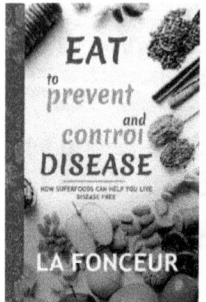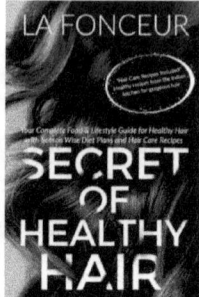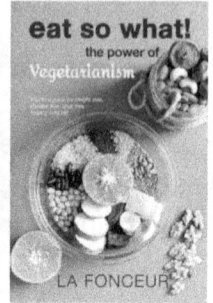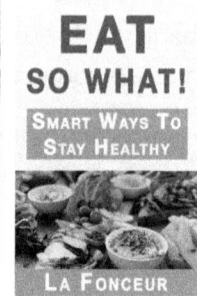

Mini extract editions:

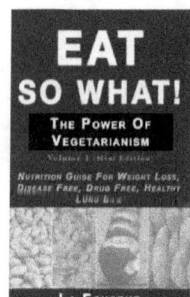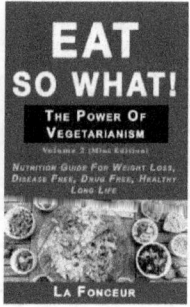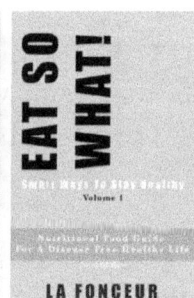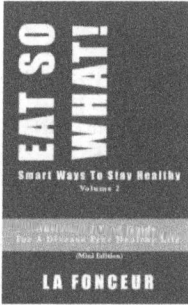

Hindi editions:

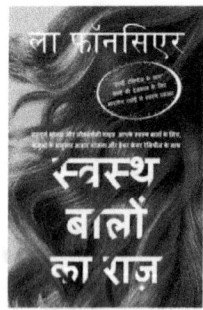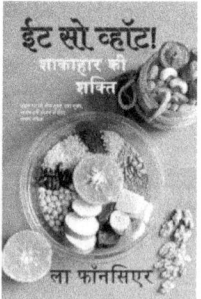

Connect with La Fonceur

Instagram: **@la_fonceur** | **@eatsowhat**

Facebook: **LaFonceur** | **eatsowhat**

Twitter: **@la_fonceur**

Amazon Author Page:

www.amazon.com/La-Fonceur/e/B07PM8SBSG/

Bookbub Author Page: **www.bookbub.com/authors/la-fonceur**

Sign up to the websites to get exclusive offers on La Fonceur eBooks:

Health Blog: **http://eatsowhat.com/esw-mailing-list/**

Website: **www.lafonceur.com/sign-up**

www.ingramcontent.com/pod-product-compliance
Lightning Source LLC
Chambersburg PA
CBHW072209170526

45158CB00002BA/517